Gross Pathology Handbook

Gross Pathology Handbook

A GUIDE TO DESCRIPTIVE TERMS

SECOND EDITION

CHRISTOPHER HORN,
MSc, PA(ASCP)CM (CCCPA-CCCAP)

CHRISTOPHER NAUGLER,
MD, MSc

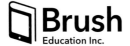

Brush Education Inc.
www.brusheducation.ca
contact@brusheducation.ca

Cover and interior design: Carol Dragich, Dragich Design

Library and Archives Canada Cataloguing in Publication

Title: Gross pathology handbook : a guide to descriptive terms / Christopher Horn, MSc, Christopher Naugler, MD, MSc.
Names: Horn, Christopher, 1972- author. | Naugler, Christopher T. (Christopher Terrance), 1967- author.
Description: Second edition. | Includes bibliographical references and index.
Identifiers: Canadiana (print) 20210279303 | Canadiana (ebook) 20210279338 | ISBN 9781550599091 (softcover) | ISBN 9781550599107 (PDF) | ISBN 9781550599114 (EPUB)
Subjects: LCSH: Anatomy, Pathological—Terminology—Handbooks, manuals, etc. | LCSH: Anatomy, Pathological—Pictorial works.
Classification: LCC RB30 .H67 2021 | DDC 616.07—dc23

We acknowledge the support of the Government of Canada
Nous reconnaissons l'appui du gouvernement du Canada | Canadä

Contents

Acknowledgements

I would like to thank Calgary Laboratory Services / Alberta Precision Labs, and in particular Dr. Jim Wright, for allowing me access to the databank of gross images for this book.

In addition, special thanks to the many pathologists, pathology residents, and gross room staff who over the years have had a role in the acquisition of these images. Thanks also to those who developed software to help organize and access them. In particular, I would like to thank Dr. Amy Bromley, Dr. Travis Ogilvie, Dr. Vincent Falck, Dammika Bambaragama, Kayla Nelson, Charity Greene, Christina Yang, Barb Scott, Arlene Dumo Cerda, Patricia McInnis, and Kristy Ells; Dr. Christopher Naugler, for recognizing the value of this project and for getting me in touch with the people at Brush Education; Bill Gorday, for reviewing the book and giving me feedback from a fellow pathologists' assistant perspective; to everyone at Brush Education, for the opportunity to publish a much needed educational resource and for keeping me on track during the process.

I dedicate this book to my wonderful children, Genevieve, Justin and Samantha.

And to my beautiful wife Dana,

Whose image needs no enhancement

— CH

Introduction

Why this guide?

As medical professionals (Christopher Horn is a pathologists' assistant, Christopher Naugler is a general pathologist and family physician), we have often wanted a resource with a comprehensive list of gross-descriptive terms and examples of gross specimens. We figured such a resource would help not only us, it would help other professionals as well: it could, for example, help standardize gross-descriptive terminology and make pathology reports more succinct.

We couldn't find a resource like this, so we created this guide.

This guide pairs a comprehensive list of gross-dissection terms with photographic examples of gross-dissection specimens.

It aims to help pathology professionals—pathology residents, pathologists' assistants, and medical laboratory technicians— describe surgical and autopsy specimens as they perform gross dissection.

The pathology gross room and autopsy suite are fascinating places that analyze specimens from the operating room. The specimens often involve a variety of disease processes, 1 or many organ systems, and—as a result—a multitude of gross appearances. Quite often, the same disease process appears different on similar specimen types, or different from patient to patient. As a pathology-lab professional, your job is to describe *what you see*, so that a pathologist or clinician can read the description and visualize the specimen. This can be a daunting task, given the variability and complexity of specimens— especially for new pathology staff at the beginning of their surgical gross-dissection training. A common question in the gross room is: "How would you describe this specimen?"

The flipside of this question, from a clinician's point of view, is: "What does this specimen look like, based on this description?" This guide also aims to help clinicians and medical students navigate pathology reports.

How to use this guide

Look up terms, look up images

If you are a lab professional who is training to perform gross surgical dissection, you can use this guide, first, as a way to study specimens and the terms to describe them. Then, as you work in the surgical gross area, you can use it to identify appropriate terms by comparing your gross findings with the images. As your skills progress, you can use it to refresh and validate your gross-descriptive skills.

As a clinician or medical student, you can use this guide "in reverse" to help interpret pathology reports: to look up unfamiliar gross-descriptive terms and see examples of specimens they describe.

Combine terms for precise description

As a lab professional, you should combine the terms in this guide as necessary to arrive at the most precise descriptions possible.

For example, to describe the appearance of a fibroid uterus, you might combine the terms *whorled* and *circumscribed*: "white-whorled, well-circumscribed masses." This description avoids words such as *fibroid* and *leiomyoma*, which are considered diagnostic terms.

Note the inclusion of some diagnostic terms

The grosser's job is to describe and the pathologist's job is to diagnose. So, gross descriptions should not, in general, employ diagnostic terminology.

We have found, however, that some diagnostic terms provide the best way to describe some gross findings, and that pathologists and clinicians often agree. This guide includes these terms.

It includes, for example, the term *diverticulum*. Although *diverticulum* is technically a diagnostic term, it is often preferred as a descriptor over the more traditional and wordy "out pouching of mucosa and intestinal wall into the surrounding pericolic fat."

You may want to check with your pathologists before incorporating these diagnostic terms into your reports.

Apply the sample gross descriptions
We use each term in this guide in a unique gross-description phrase, usually based on the specimen in the accompanying image.

You can use these phrases as the foundation of your own reporting.

Disclaimer
The publisher, authors, contributors, and editors bring substantial expertise to this reference and have made their best efforts to ensure that it is useful, accurate, safe, and reliable.

Nonetheless, practitioners must always rely on their own expertise, knowledge, and judgment when consulting any of the information contained in this reference or employing it in patient care. When using any of this information, they should remain conscious of their responsibility for their own safety and the safety of others, and for the best interests of those in their care.

To the fullest extent of the law, neither the publishers, the authors, the contributors, nor the editors assume any liability for injury or damage to persons from any use of information or ideas contained in this reference.

Abrasion

Gross appearance and identification
An irregular skin defect, or scraped area of the skin
- It is an injury caused by superficial damage to the skin, no deeper than the epidermis.
- Scarring does not usually occur, due to the superficial nature of the wound.

Tissues commonly affected
Skin

Common etiology
Usually occurs due to traumatic injury

Sample gross description
"Present on the surface is a focal, irregular **abrasion** measuring . . . "

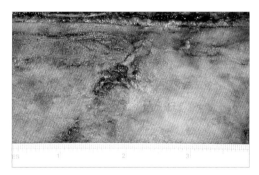

An abrasion caused by trauma

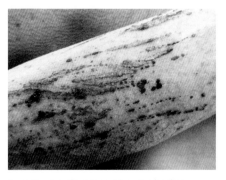

An extensive abrasion with some healing

Adhesion

Gross appearance and identification
Opaque light-tan or gray-tan fibrous bands of scar tissue that form between internal organs and tissues, joining them together abnormally
- Adhesions are made up of connective tissue cells that form as a normal part of the body's healing process and help to limit the spread of infection.
- They are commonly seen in perforated specimens and as a result of previous surgery.

Tissues commonly affected
Loops of the intestines; the intestines and other abdominal organs or the abdominal wall; abdominal organs such as the liver or bladder and the abdominal wall; tissues of the uterus

Common etiology
Asherman syndrome, postsurgical complications

Sample gross description
"The distal end of the small bowel has folded over and become **adherent** to itself . . . "

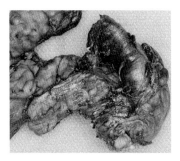

A large bowel segment that has looped around and become adherent to itself as a result of a perforation

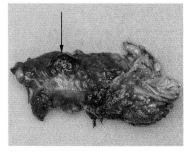

An adherent mucinous tumor on the outer surface of the bowel

Annular/circinate

Gross appearance and identification
A lesion or area of interest that is shaped like, or forms, a ring
- An annular lesion likely indicates an inflammatory process or a malignant process.

Tissues commonly affected
Mucous membranes, skin

Common etiology
Colonic adenocarcinoma, dermatophytosis, sarcoidosis, tinea

Sample gross description
"Present on the mucosal surface is an **annular/circinate** elevated lesion measuring . . . "

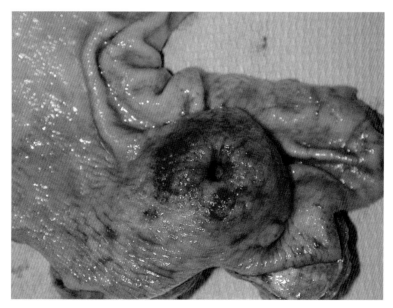

An annular lesion present in the colonic mucosa

Anthracotic pigment

Gross appearance and identification
Black diffuse pigmentation on the surface of a specimen
- Anthracosis is an accumulation of carbon pigment from breathing dirty air or smoke.
- Smokers have the most pronounced anthracosis, but it can be seen in the majority of urban dwellers.

Tissues commonly affected
Lungs, mediastinal lymph nodes

Common etiology
Smoking, living in urban areas with high levels of pollution

Sample gross description
"The external surface appears mostly smooth with diffuse **anthracotic pigmentation . . .** "

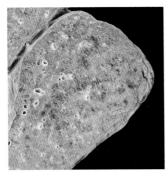

Diffuse anthracotic pigmentation on the cut surface of a lung

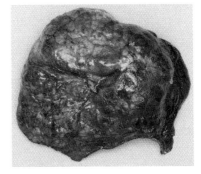

Diffuse anthracotic pigmentation on the surface of a lung

Apple-core

Gross appearance and identification
A relatively short, sharply defined lesion of circumferential, annular, constricting colonic narrowing with overhanging margins
- Most commonly, this lesion is an adenocarcinoma arising in the large intestine, but can present as a tumor in the esophagus.

Tissues commonly affected
Large intestine, small intestine, esophagus

Common etiology
Adenocarcinoma

Sample gross description
"Present on the mucosal surface of the large intestine is a well-circumscribed, raised, **apple-core** lesion measuring . . . "

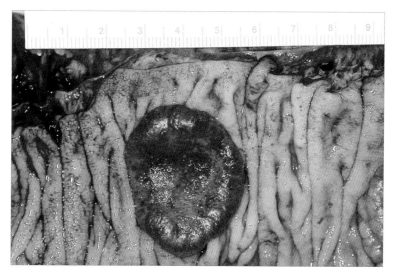

An apple-core lesion present in the mucosa of the large intestine

Asymmetrical

Gross appearance and identification
A lesion, organ, or area of interest that lacks symmetry
- Asymmetrical specimens exhibit dissimilarity in corresponding, normally similar parts or organs on opposite sides of the body.

Tissues commonly affected
Any organ or tissue that is bilateral or has right-left hemispheres

Common etiology
Any disease process including tumors, inflammation, and edema

Sample gross description
"The specimen consists of a total thyroidectomy specimen with **asymmetrical** lobes."

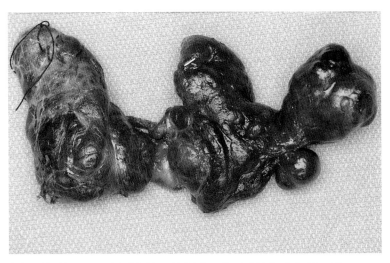

A thyroid with asymmetrical right and left lobes: the right lobe (left side of the photograph, with the stitch), appears normal; the left lobe is more lobulated and irregular

Atelectatic

Gross appearance and identification and identification
A collapse of lung tissue affecting part or all of a lung
- Blockages can occur due to a mucous "plug," foreign object, or tumor, or because of a surgical complication. When a blockage occurs, the alveoli are unable to fill with air: collapse of lung tissue can occur in the affected area.
- This condition may be localized or may affect all of both lungs.

Tissues commonly affected
Lungs

Common etiology
Tumors, mucous "plugs," foreign objects, congenital atelectasis

Sample gross description
"The specimen has an **atelectatic** appearance affecting one-half of the specimen."

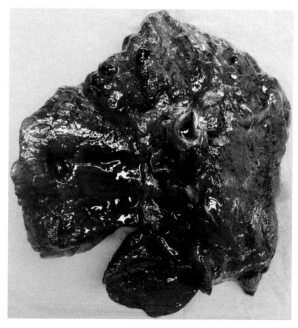

A lung that is atelectatic (collapsed) on the left side, due to a tumor obstruction located near the bronchus

Atrophic

Gross appearance and identification
A wasting or decrease in size of a body organ, tissue, or part owing to injury, disease, or lack of use

Tissues commonly affected
Any

Common etiology
Amyotrophia, amyotrophy, kraurosis, cachexia, muscular dystrophy

Sample gross description
"The right kidney appears **atrophic** and measures . . . "

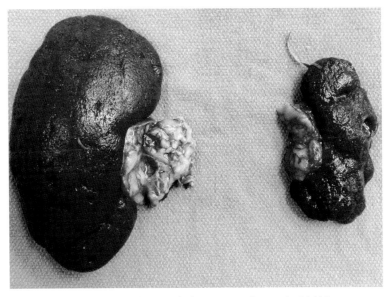

An atrophic kidney (on the right): a pathologic process has made this kidney markedly decreased in size (atrophic) compared to the normal-appearing kidney on the left

Bilateral

Gross appearance and identification
Any gross appearance involving both the left and right sides of
the body
- *Bilateral* refers to paired organs that are on opposite sides of
  the body, such as kidneys, parotid glands, etc.
- The term can also be used to describe conditions and
  procedures that affect both body sides: for example, *bilateral
  mastectomy*.

Tissues commonly affected
Any organ that exhibits bilateral symmetry such as the kidneys,
adrenal glands, thyroid, ovaries, and lungs

Common etiology
Pulmonary embolism, thyroiditis, polycystic kidney disease,
arthritis, Addison disease

Sample gross description
"The specimen consists of hysterectomy and attached **bilateral**
salpingo-oophorectomy."

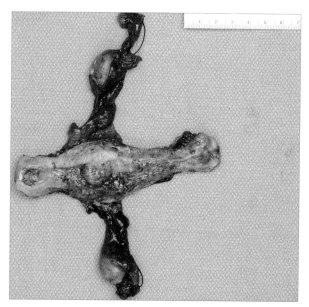

Hysterectomy specimen with attached bilateral salpingo-
oophorectomy

Bile-stained

Gross appearance and identification
A green to dark-green fluid that is absorbed into the lining or mucosa of a specimen
  • Bile originates in the liver, and is concentrated and stored in the gallbladder.

Tissues commonly affected
Gall bladder, small intestine, peritoneal cavity, stomach

Common etiology
Gall bladder mucosa (normal finding) or liver disease if found in the peritoneal cavity

Sample gross description
"The mucosa is granular and **bile-stained** . . . "

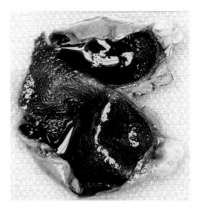

A gallbladder with green bile staining on the mucosa

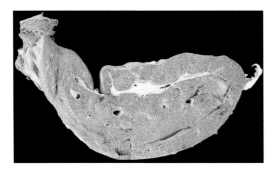

Bile staining on the cut surface of a liver

Bivalved

Gross appearance and identification
A specimen cut into 2 equal parts
- Bivalving is usually done in the pathology lab: specimens are generally sent intact to the lab.
- It is done to examine the internal contents of specimens, or to facilitate formalin fixation of pathologic specimens.

Tissues commonly affected
Any tissue removed from the body and sent to the pathology lab

Common etiology
N/A

Sample gross description
"The specimen is received intact and is **bivalved** to reveal . . . "

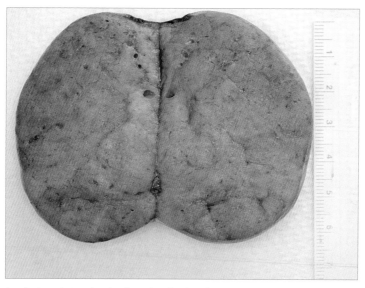

A soft-tissue lesion that has been bivalved to show the cut surface

Blister

Gross appearance and identification
A localized swelling of the skin that contains watery fluid
- Blisters are saccular skin vesicles filled with serous fluid that separate the epidermis and/or dermis, and that can arise from trauma, burns, or vesicatory agents.

Tissues commonly affected
Skin, mucosa

Common etiology
Trauma, burning, infection, or irritation

Sample gross description
"Present on the plantar surface is a dark-red **blister** measuring . . . "

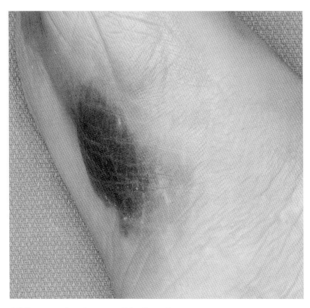

A blister on the dorsum of the foot due to trauma

Bosselated

Gross appearance and identification
An area marked by numerous bosses or rounded protuberances
- *Bosselated* is usually reserved for describing the surface of specimens.
- Underlying tumors are usually responsible for bosselated areas.

Tissues commonly affected
Skin; serosal and organ surfaces

Common etiology
Malignant or benign tumors, leiomyomas, edema

Sample gross description
"The surface of the specimen is smooth with a **bosselated** appearance."

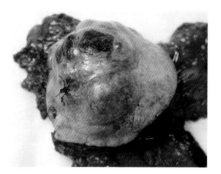

A skin surface that is bosselated due to an underlying tumor

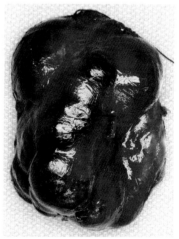

An external surface that is bosselated due to an underlying disease process

Botryoid

Gross appearance and identification
Numerous rounded protuberances
- The protuberances can be fluid-filled cystic structures or solid.
- They are usually translucent or transparent.
- They resemble "a bunch of grapes."

Tissues commonly affected
Soft tissue tumors, molar pregnancies, polyps

Common etiology
Molar pregnancy, odontogenic cyst, sarcoma botryoides (botryoid sarcoma, botryoid rhabdomyosarcoma)

Sample gross description
"The cyst is opened to reveal that it is filled with multiple **botryoid** cysts ranging in size from . . . "

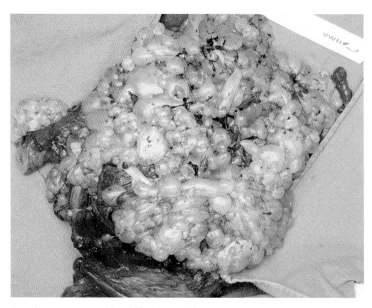

A molar pregnancy with a diffuse botryoid appearance

Bulla

Gross appearance and identification

A large vesicle or blister (> 5 mm in diameter)

- Bullas are similar to blisters in contents and appearance, but larger.
- The term is often used to describe thin-walled balloon-like extensions or air sacs that are commonly found in lungs.

Tissues commonly affected

Skin, lung

Common etiology

In the skin, trauma; in the lung, emphysema, chronic obstructive pulmonary disease (COPD), or spontaneous pneumothorax

Sample gross description

"Present on the surface is a single, transparent **bulla** measuring . . . "

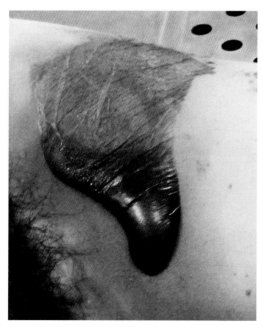

A bulla filled with bloody fluid present on a skin surface

Calculus

Gross appearance and identification
Firm, stone-like objects that occupy lumens or ducts
- Calculi are usually found in biliary and urinary tracts.
- Calculi are abnormal stones formed in body tissues by an accumulation of mineral salts.

Tissues commonly affected
Gallbladder, kidneys

Common etiology
Cholelithiasis, renal calculi

Sample gross description
"The gallbladder contains a single, firm dark-tan, ovoid **calculus** measuring . . . "

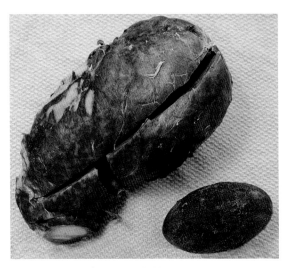

An ovoid calculus from a gallbladder

Caseous

Gross appearance and identification
A necrotic lesion or area of interest that is cottage cheese–like in appearance

Tissues commonly affected
Lung

Common etiology
Infections such as tuberculosis; central necrosis in malignant tumors

Sample gross description
"The cystic cavity contains **caseous** and necrotic material."

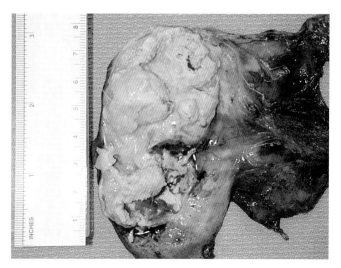

A lesion with a classic caseous and necrotic appearance

Centrally located

Gross appearance and identification
A lesion or landmark that occupies the central space of a specimen

Tissues commonly affected
Any

Common etiology
N/A

Sample gross description
"Present on the skin ellipse is a **centrally located**, everted nipple measuring . . . "

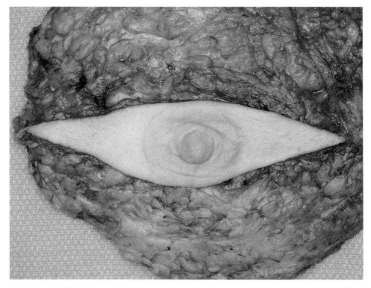

A nipple that is centrally located because it appears in the middle of the skin ellipse

Chalky

Gross appearance and identification

An opaque tan or white-tan soft material occupying spaces or surfaces in a specimen

- *Chalky* is also often used to describe the unique gross features of a person with gout.
- Chalky material usually indicates defective calcification or fatty necrosis.

Tissues commonly affected

Toes, soft tissues, teeth

Common etiology

Gout, chronic pancreatitis, onychomycosis, tumoral calcinosis

Sample gross description

"The cut surface reveals an irregular pattern of **chalky** material . . . "

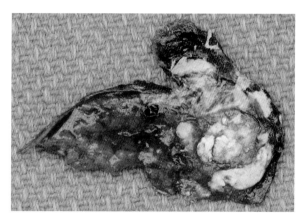

A specimen containing chalky material due to gout

Circular/donut-shaped

Gross appearance and identification
A lesion or specimen that is circular and hollow
- *Circular/donut-shaped* can be used to refer to the shape of a lesion or the shape of a whole specimen.

Tissues commonly affected
Any

Common etiology
N/A

Sample gross description
"The specimen consists of a **circular/donut-shaped** portion of colonic mucosa measuring . . . "

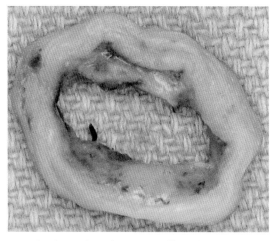

A circular/donut-shaped specimen of large bowel, exhibiting all of the mucosal and muscular layers

Circumferential

Gross appearance and identification
A lesion or area of interest that is encircling and/or pertains to
a circumference or perimeter of a specimen
- *Circumferential* is often reserved for gross descriptions of
  luminal specimens, such as the intestinal tract.

Tissues commonly affected
Luminal structures, such as the gastrointestinal (GI) tract

Common etiology
Tumors, objects causing obstruction

Sample gross description
"Present in the midportion of the large intestine is an
ulcerating, **circumferential** neoplasm measuring . . . "

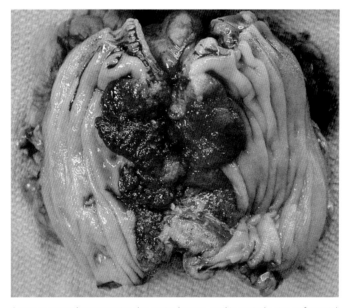

A tumor mass that occupies the entire lumen, and is entirely circumferential

Circumscribed

Gross appearance and identification
A lesion or structure contained in a well-defined area, or within definite boundaries or limits

- *Circumscribed* is usually used to describe the appearance of a lesion within a specimen.
- Well-circumscribed lesions are often benign.

Tissues commonly affected
Any

Common etiology
Lipoma, adenomas, leiomyomas

Sample gross description
"The cut surface reveals an ovoid, well-**circumscribed**, yellow, homogeneous lesion measuring . . . "

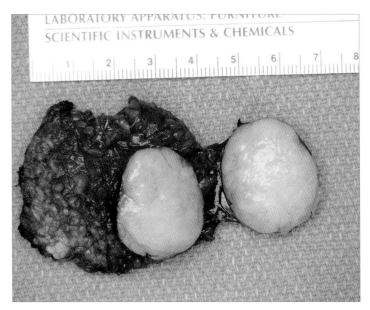

A well-circumscribed mass in a portion of surgically removed subcutaneous tissue

Clot/thrombus

Gross appearance and identification
Dark-red, soft, insoluble, jellylike masses
- Clots are formed when blood or lymph coagulates.
- Abnormal blood clots can cause heart attack, stroke, or other serious medical issues.

Tissues commonly affected
Vessels, major organ systems

Common etiology
Deep vein thrombosis, stroke, myocardial infarction, thrombosis

Sample gross description
"The specimen is bivalved to reveal a dilated renal calyx containing a blood **clot/thrombus** measuring . . . "

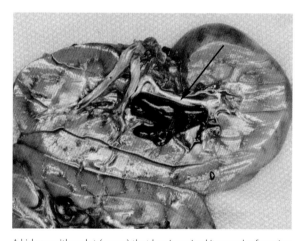

A kidney with a clot (arrow) that has impaired its regular function

Coalesced

Gross appearance and identification
A lesion with 2 or more areas adherent or attached to each
other due to a pathologic process
- Coalesced lesions have a joining or fusing of parts.
- In pathology, coalescing is commonly observed as numerous
  raised nodules that often appear in groups on the skin
  surface of the knees, elbows, and lower extremities. The
  nodules coalesce to form a large patch that appears to be a
  single lesion.

Tissues commonly affected
Any area affected by multifocal disease

Common etiology
Tumors; benign or malignant skin lesions

Sample gross description
"The cut surface shows 2 white, well-circumscribed lesions that
have **coalesced** to form a larger lesion measuring . . . "

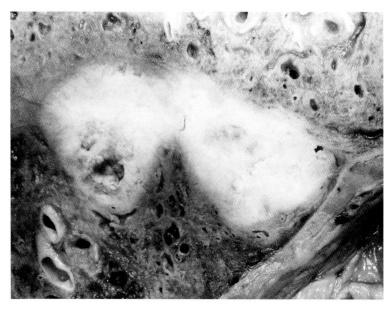

Lung lesions that have come together in a coalescing appearance

Cobblestone

Gross appearance and identification
A morphology or pattern characterized by multiple, similarly sized, rounded densities, which project from a single linear surface that rises above a flattened plane
- A typical example of cobblestoning arises from uniform nodules, due to submucosal edema, with crisscrossing of the ulcers through inflamed but intact intestinal mucosa.

Tissues commonly affected
GI tract

Common etiology
Crohn disease, ulcerative colitis

Sample gross description
"The mucosal surface of the large intestine exhibits a **cobblestone** pattern . . . "

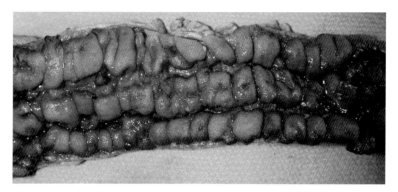

A typical cobblestone pattern due to Crohn disease

Congested

Gross appearance and identification

A lesion or area of interest with dark-blue to purple tissue

- Congested tissue is characterized by an excessive accumulation of a substance such as blood. Congestion may result from increased production of the substance and/or flow of the substance into the tissue.

- Congestion also can result from a decreased ability of the heart to pump, leading to lung congestion.

Tissues commonly affected

Any

Common etiology

Infarct, torsion

Sample gross description

"There is a well-circumscribed, ovoid, deeply **congested** mass attached to the fallopian tube measuring . . . "

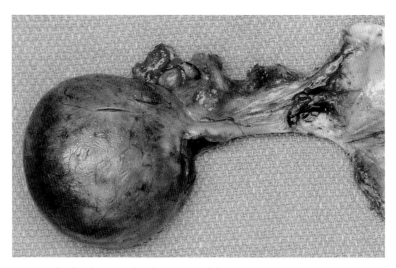

An ovary that has become deeply congested due to torsion

Corrugated

Gross appearance and identification
A lesion or area of interest that has folds, or parallel and
alternating ridges and grooves

Tissues commonly affected
Any

Common etiology
Trauma

Sample gross description
"The skull has been previously fractured in a **corrugated** pattern,
with the fracture site measuring . . . "

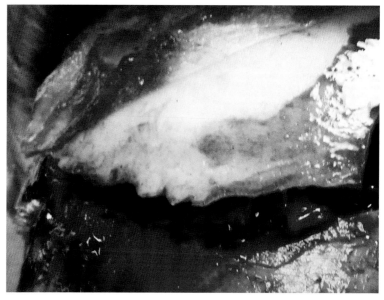

A portion of skull showing a corrugated pattern of fractures, with alternating and
parallel ridges and grooves

Crystalline

Gross appearance and identification
A lesion or area of interest that is transparent, and appears composed of mineral, glass, or crystal

- The appearance comes from plane faces intersecting at definite angles.
- Crystalline appearance is often associated with calculi or crystal-forming diseases.

Tissues commonly affected
Gallbladder, kidney

Common etiology
Cholelithiasis, kidney stones

Sample gross description
"The lumen contains a **crystalline** calculus measuring . . . "

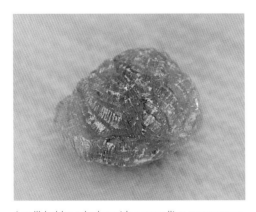

A gallbladder calculus with a crystalline appearance

Cylindrical

Gross appearance and identification
A lesion or gross appearance that relates to, or has the shape of, a cylinder, especially of a circular cylinder
- In the body, there are many structures that have a lumen and are referred to as cylindrical in shape.

Tissues commonly affected
Appendix, fallopian tube, vas deferens

Common etiology
N/A

Sample gross description
"The specimen consists of a single, soft-tan **cylindrical** portion of tissue measuring . . . "

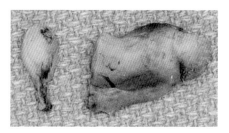

A fallopian tube with a typical, cylindrical appearance; the section on the left (a cross section) shows the lumen

Cystic

Gross appearance and identification
An abnormal membranous sac containing a gaseous, liquid, or semisolid substance

Tissues commonly affected
Any, but most commonly ovaries and skin

Common etiology
Ovarian cysts, dermoid cysts, blood cysts, hydatid, pilar cysts, sebaceous cysts

Sample gross description
"The mass is incised to reveal a **cystic** cavity containing . . . "

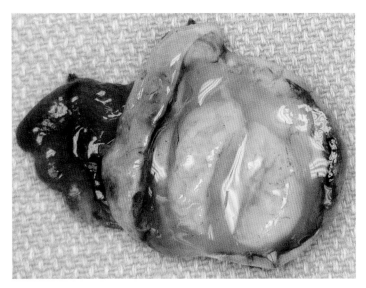

A cyst with both a liquid and semisolid appearance

Defect

Gross appearance and identification
An imperfection or hole in a specimen
- Defects are usually associated with trauma or surgery.

Tissues commonly affected
Any

Common etiology
Trauma

Sample gross description
"Present on the anterior serosal surface is a focal, irregular **defect** measuring . . . "

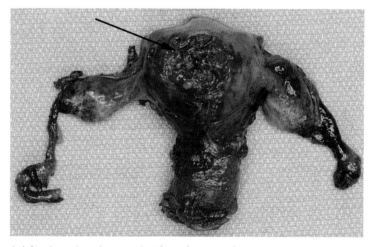

A defect (arrow) on the serosal surface of a uterine fundus (a tear created during surgical removal of the specimen)

Degeneration

Gross appearance and identification
Necrosis; or areas of solid, uninvolved tissue with central or peripheral necrosis

- Degeneration is often seen grossly in large tumor masses that have outgrown their blood supply.
- Degeneration is the hallmark of tissues, cells, or organs with gradual deterioration, impairment, or loss of function, caused by injury, disease, or aging.

Tissues commonly affected
Any

Common etiology
Malignant tumors, areas with decreased vascular supply

Sample gross description
"The specimen is bivalved to reveal a well-circumscribed neoplasm with central, cystic **degeneration**."

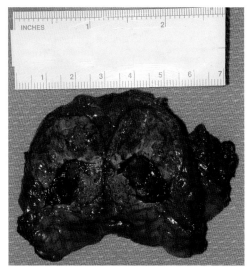

A malignant tumor with central, cystic degeneration from outgrowing its blood supply

Demarcated

Gross appearance and identification
A lesion or area of interest that shows a sharp transition from one gross appearance to another
  • The transition may occur from a disease process to normal tissue.

Tissues commonly affected
Any, but most commonly seen in the GI tract

Common etiology
Ischemia, inflammatory bowel disease

Sample gross description
"The small intestine mucosa exhibits grossly normal mucosal folding and light-tan color with a sharply **demarcated** transition into congested mucosa located . . . "

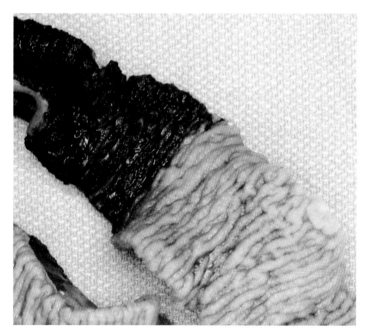

A sharp demarcation between hemorrhagic colon mucosa and normal-appearing bowel mucosa

Dense/solid

Gross appearance and identification
A compact structure, containing no hollow or liquid-filled pockets

- Often, tissues can present as dense or solid due to a desmoplastic response to chronic inflammation and/or tumors.
- Both benign and malignant tumors can have a solid appearance.

Tissues commonly affected
Any, but commonly breast and colon

Common etiology
Chronic inflammation, tumors, desmoplastic response, fibrothecoma, fibroids, fibroma, fibromatosis

Sample gross description
"The specimen is bivalved to reveal a **dense/solid** heterogeneous yellow and fibrous cut surface."

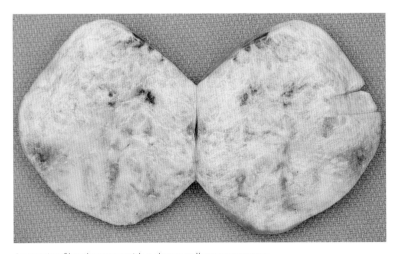

An ovarian fibrothecoma with a dense, yellow appearance

Depressed

Gross appearance and identification
An area of interest that exhibits a hollow area with downward or inward displacement
- A depression may indicate a disease process such as edema, where an indentation is produced by pressure.

Tissues commonly affected
Any, but most commonly subcutaneous tissues

Common etiology
Pitting edema

Sample gross description
"The specimen exhibits an overall edematous appearance with a focal **depressed** area located superior to the second knuckle on the fourth digit."

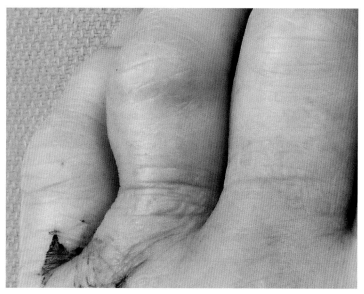

A focal depression below the middle digit of a patient's hand, due to edema in the extremities and a (now removed) ring

Diffuse

Gross appearance and identification
A disease process that is spread out or distributed across a specimen
- A diffuse distribution of a lesion may indicate local metastasis in malignant lesions.

Tissues commonly affected
Any

Common etiology
Malignant tumors, infectious diseases (e.g., tuberculosis)

Sample gross description
"The cut surface of this lesion shows normal liver parenchyma with a background of **diffuse** grey-tan tumor."

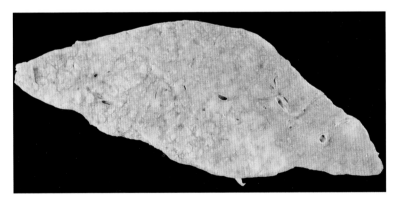

A diffuse pattern of malignancy in a cut surface of a liver

Dilated

Gross appearance and identification
A widening or expansion of a particular area in a specimen
- *Dilated* is usually reserved for luminal structures of the body, including vessels and areas of the GI tract.
- Dilation can arise from increased vascular flow in vessels or obstructions in luminal structures.

Tissues commonly affected
GI tract, vessels, fallopian tubes

Common etiology
Emphysema, obstructions due to clots, inflammation, tumors, etc.

Sample gross description
"The cut surface of the specimen shows multiple **dilated** vessels ranging in diameter from . . . "

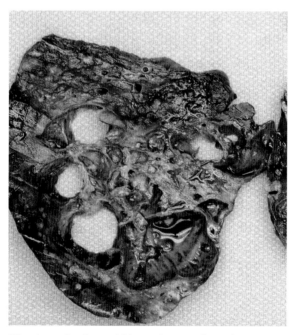

Dilated areas in a lung, which are air sacs and vessels

Discoloration

Gross appearance and identification
An alteration in color from normal appearance
  • Discoloration can arise from a variety of disease processes—
    for example, tumors and infarcts of vasculature.

Tissues commonly affected
Any

Common etiology
Ischemia, infarct

Sample gross description
"The surface appears smooth and mostly yellow with a focal area of dark-red **discoloration** measuring . . . "

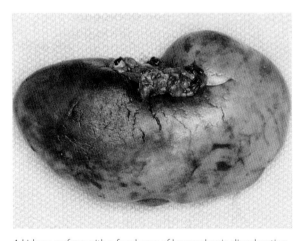

A kidney surface with a focal area of hemorrhagic discoloration

Distended

Gross appearance and identification
Stretching or swelling in a specimen caused by internal pressure

Tissues commonly affected
GI tract

Common etiology
Bowel obstruction, aneurism, arteriovenous malformation

Sample gross description
"Present at the midportion of the large intestine is a **distended** area measuring . . . "

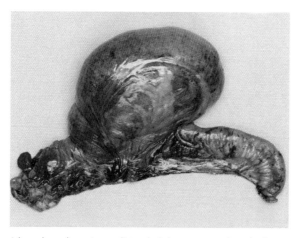

A large bowel specimen distended due to trapped gas in the lumen, causing expansion of the luminal space and stretching of the bowel wall

Diverticulum

Gross appearance and identification
An outpouching of a hollow (or a fluid-filled) structure
- Diverticula can affect many or all of the layers of the structure involved.
- Severe diverticular disease can cause perforations, resulting in abscesses and bleeding, especially in the colon.

Tissues commonly affected
GI tract, urethra, bladder, gallbladder, appendix

Common etiology
Diverticulitis

Sample gross description
"The distal tip of the appendix, which does not appear perforated, is sectioned to reveal prominent **diverticula**."

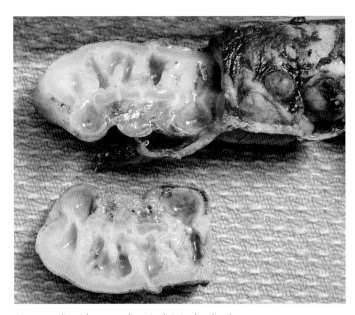

An appendix with severe diverticulitis in the distal aspect

Eccentrically located

Gross appearance and identification
A lesion or gross finding that is off center

- In gross pathology, *eccentrically located* is often used to describe the appearance of a lesion in relation to the rest of the specimen.

Tissues commonly affected
Any organ

Common etiology
Tumor masses and other lesions

Sample gross description
"The capsular surface is mostly smooth and unremarkable except for a focal, well-circumscribed, **eccentrically located** raised lesion measuring . . . "

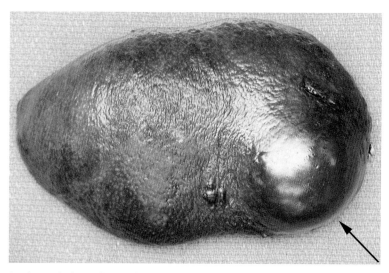

A subcapsular lesion (arrow) that is eccentrically located (off center)

Edematous

Gross appearance and identification
A swelling of otherwise normal-appearing tissue
- The swelling arises from an abnormal accumulation of fluid in the interstitium, which is located beneath the skin, or in 1 or more cavities of the body.

Tissues commonly affected
Cutaneous tissues, GI tract

Common etiology
Cutaneous edema, pulmonary edema, peripheral edema

Sample gross description
"The distal aspect of the large bowel appears mostly **edematous** with a focal area of necrosis measuring . . . "

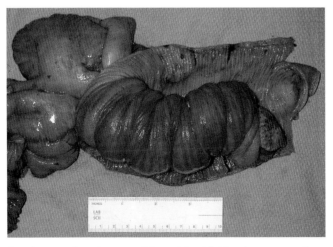

An edematous bowel mucosa: it has retained fluid and appears swollen

Ellipse

Gross appearance and identification

A specimen shaped like an ellipse

- The term *ellipse* is reserved in pathology for describing the general shape of some specimens.
- An ellipse is a common shape in skin excision specimens, such as wide excisions for skin cancer, and in breast mastectomy specimens.

Tissues commonly affected

Skin

Common specimen sources

Skin cancers and underlying disease processes where skin excision is needed; mastectomy specimens

Sample gross description

"The specimen consists of a tan **ellipse** of skin with underlying subcutaneous tissue measuring . . . "

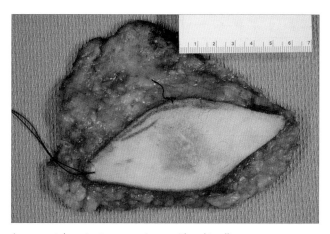

A segmental mastectomy specimen with a skin ellipse

Elongated

Gross appearance and identification

Tissue or structures that appear stretched out compared to normal

- *Elongated* is reserved for describing specimens in comparison to the normal appearance of the specimen.
- Note that elongated appearance does not necessarily indicate any underlying disease process.

Tissues commonly affected

Any

Common etiology

N/A

Sample gross description

"The fallopian tube is present and appears **elongated**, measuring . . . "

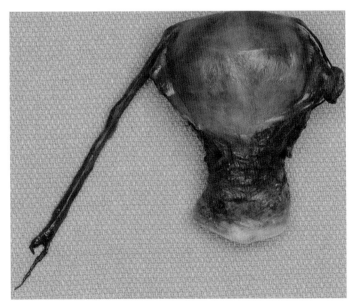

A fallopian tube that appears stretched out (elongated)

Encapsulated

Gross appearance and identification
A space enclosed by a coating or membrane
- In general, *encapsulated* refers to a tumor confined to a specific area, surrounded by a thin layer of fibrous tissue.
- Lesions with protective capsules are often benign.

Tissues commonly affected
Any, but most commonly thyroid, breast, ovaries, lipoma

Common etiology
Follicular lesions of the thyroid, ovarian tumors

Sample gross description
"The specimen is bivalved to reveal a well-circumscribed, ovoid, **encapsulated** cystic lesion measuring . . . "

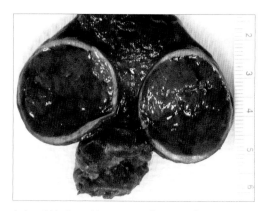

A thyroid lesion with a surrounding capsule

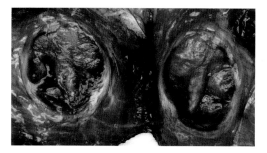

Another example of an encapsulated thyroid lesion

Encircling

Gross appearance and identification

A lesion or area of interest that forms a circle around, or
surrounds, another area or structure

- Circumferential colon cancers have been grossly described
  as *encircling*.

Tissues commonly affected

Any, but most commonly skin

Common etiology

Infections, trauma, colon cancer

Sample gross description

"The specimen consists of a portion of skin that has 2 focal
circular defects with distinct red **encircling** areas surrounding
the orifices measuring . . . "

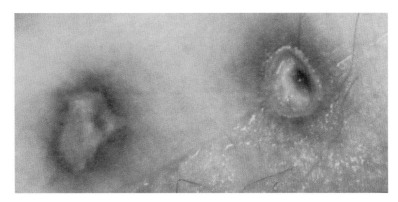

Skin lesions showing an encircling red inflammatory reaction at the skin surface

Eroded

Gross appearance and identification
A wearing away of overlying tissue
- Erosions appear as slightly depressed areas of skin in which part or all of the epidermis has been lost.
- They are generally due to chronic trauma, neoplasia, or inflammation.

Tissues commonly affected
Skin

Common etiology
Trauma, neoplasia, chronic inflammation

Sample gross description
"Present on the skin surface is a focal, well-defined, **eroded** lesion measuring . . . "

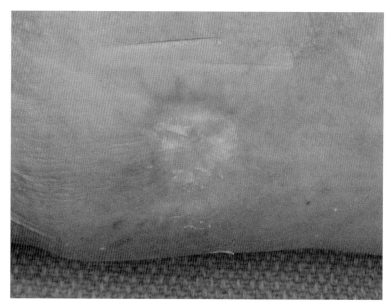

A superficial epidermal layer that has been eroded by trauma

Everted

Gross appearance and identification
An area or lesion on a specimen that protrudes outward compared to the rest of the specimen

Tissues commonly affected
Skin

Common etiology
N/A

Sample gross description
"Present on the skin surface is a centrally located, **everted** nipple measuring . . . "

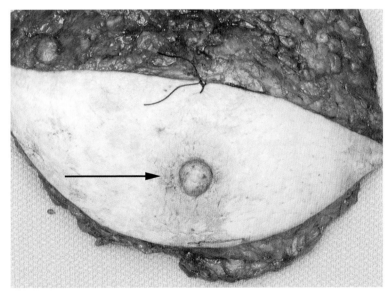

A skin ellipse with a centrally located nipple (arrow), which is everted (protruding outward from the skin surface)

Excoriated

Gross appearance and identification
A lesion or area of interest of the skin that has undergone a
superficial abrading or wearing off

- Excoriation can occur as an injury to a surface of the
  body caused by trauma, such as scratching, abrasion, or a
  chemical or thermal burn.

Tissues commonly affected
Skin

Common etiology
Trauma, chemical burns, thermal burns

Sample gross description
"Present on the skin surface is a focal, ill-defined **excoriated**-
appearing lesion measuring . . . "

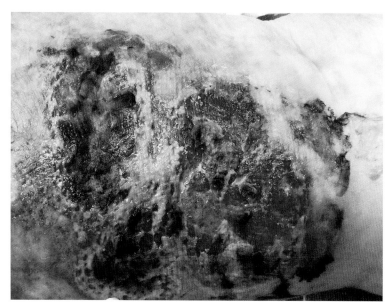

A skin surface with a focal excoriated appearance due to a traumatic injury

Excrescence

Gross appearance and identification
An abnormal outgrowth or projection related to a disease or pathologic condition
- The presence of excrescences in a specimen may indicate a premalignant or malignant condition.

Tissues commonly affected
Ovaries

Common etiology
Borderline ovarian tumors

Sample gross description
"The opened cyst reveals an internal lining containing diffuse papillary **excrescences** ranging in size from . . . "

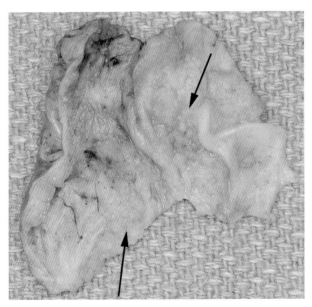

Papillary excrescences (arrows) emanating from the inner ovarian lining

Exophytic

Gross appearance and identification

An outgrowth, often lobulated or irregular in appearance

- Exophytic lesions grow outward from a surface and can be seen almost anywhere in the body.

Tissues commonly affected

Skin, liver, kidney, oral mucosa

Common etiology

Tumors

Sample gross description

"Present on the skin surface is a dark-tan and grey-tan raised, **exophytic** lesion measuring . . . "

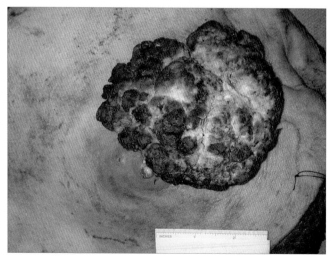

An exophytic lesion arising from breast tissue with an underlying cancer: the cancer has infiltrated the skin surface and grown outward

Exudate

Gross appearance and identification

An opaque, soft, light-tan or gray-tan material that is adherent to the surface of a specimen

- Exudate is a fluid with a high content of protein and cellular debris that has escaped from blood vessels, and been deposited in tissues or on tissue surfaces.
- It is usually a result of inflammation.

Tissues commonly affected

Appendix, bowel, peritoneal surfaces, other abdominal organs

Common etiology

Appendicitis, bowel perforation, peritonitis

Sample gross description

"Present on the distal tip is attached **exudate** measuring . . . "

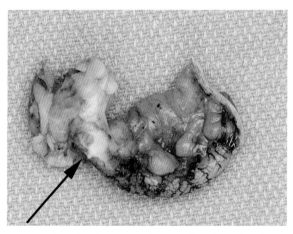

An appendix with adherent purulent exudates (arrow) at the distal tip

Fat necrosis

Gross appearance and identification
Small (1 to 4 mm), dull, chalky, gray or white foci
- Classified as the death of adipose tissue, fat necrosis is characterized by the formation of minute quantities of calcium soaps formed in the affected tissue when fat is hydrolyzed into glycerol and fatty acids.

Tissues commonly affected
Pancreas, breast, subcutaneous tissue

Common etiology
Hemorrhagic pancreatitis, trauma, collagen vascular disease, myeloproliferative disorders

Sample gross description
"The cut surface reveals a heterogeneous, lobulated lesion with focal areas of possible **fat necrosis** . . . "

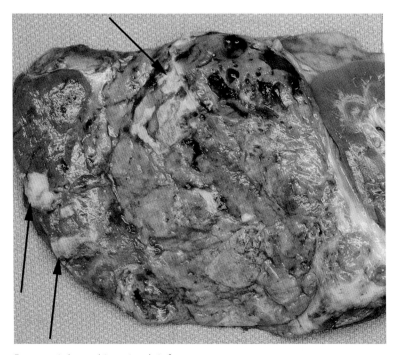

Fat necrosis (arrows) in perinephric fat

Fenestrated

Gross appearance and identification
A lesion or area of interest that has window-like openings
- The openings in fenestrated specimens can occur naturally or may be surgically created (e.g., an opening in a biological membrane).

Tissues commonly affected
Trachea, arteries, oral cavity

Common etiology
Surgical perforation of the mucoperiosteum, fenestrated tracheal defect, trauma

Sample gross description
"There are 2 **fenestrated** lesions on the lateral and posterior portion of the leg measuring . . . "

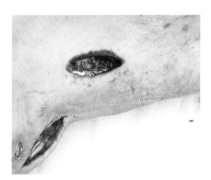

A leg with surgically created fenestrated openings that expose the subcutaneous tissues, muscle, and bone

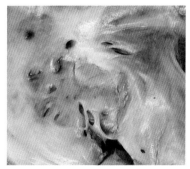

A fenestrated lesion in the foramen ovale of a heart

Fibrofatty

Gross appearance and identification
Yellow, lobulated tissue with gray-white tissue bands throughout
- *Fibrofatty* specifically refers to tissue that contains both fibrous and fatty components.
- Fibrofatty tissue is usually normal in subcutaneous tissues, and is mostly found in the breast.

Tissues commonly affected
Breast, subcutaneous tissue

Common etiology
N/A

Sample gross description
"Sectioning the specimen reveals a **fibrofatty** cut surface, with no focal lesions . . . "

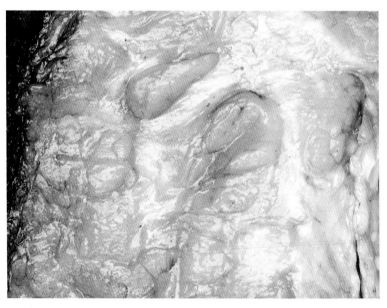

Fibrofatty tissue in a breast

Fibrous

Gross appearance and identification

Dense white to gray homogeneous or striated tissue

- Fibrous tissue consists of the common connective tissue of the body, composed of yellow or white parallel elastic and collagen fibers.

Tissues commonly affected

Breast and other soft tissues

Common etiology

Fibromatosis, fibrous dysplasia, fibroma

Sample gross description

"The specimen is sectioned to reveal a mostly **fibrous** cut surface with a focal soft, yellow, lobulated area."

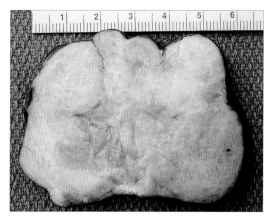

A soft-tissue tumor almost entirely composed of dense fibrous tissue with a striated appearance

Filiform

Gross appearance and identification

A lesion or area of interest that forms or resembles a thread or filament
- A filiform gross appearance can be normal, but can also indicate a disease process.

Tissues commonly affected

Skin

Common etiology

Viral warts, some cancers, normal heart structures

Sample gross description

"The specimen is sectioned to reveal a normal muscular and **filiform** appearance."

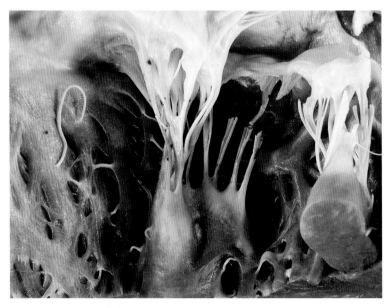

A heart with a normal filiform appearance on sectioning

Firm

Gross appearance and identification
Areas of tissue, or an entire tissue specimen, with a solid, almost unyielding surface or structure
- Most tissue specimens received in the pathology lab are soft in consistency, so variations from this norm are described as "firm" or having "firmness" in comparison to other tissues.

Tissues commonly affected
Calcified areas

Common etiology
Calciphylaxis

Sample gross description
"The specimen is sectioned to reveal a mostly yellow, lobulated cut surface with a focal, ill-defined **firm**, possibly calcified area measuring . . . "

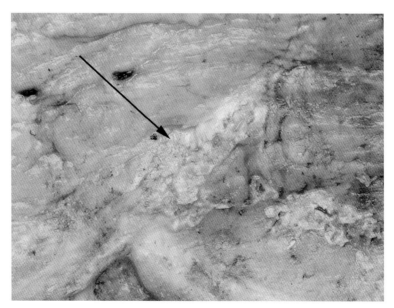

A focal area of firm calcification (arrow) contained within a soft tissue tumor

Fistula

Gross appearance and identification
An abnormal connection between 2 organs, or between an organ and the exterior of the body
- Fistulas can develop in any part of the body.
- They are most common in the digestive tract, between blood vessels, and in the urinary, reproductive, and lymphatic systems.
- Congenital conditions and a number of pathologic processes can lead to the formation of fistulas.

Tissues commonly affected
GI tract, urinary tract, reproductive tract

Common etiology
Inflammatory bowel disease, diabetes, AIDS, cancer

Sample gross description
"The specimen is sectioned to reveal a **fistula** that appears to connect the . . . "

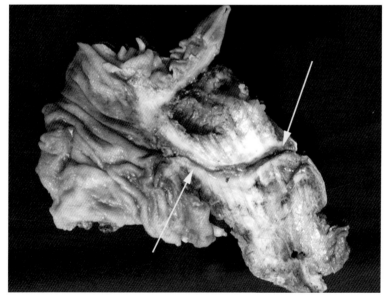

A fistula (arrows) connecting the large bowel with vaginal mucosa

Flat

Gross appearance and identification
Smooth and even, without marked lumps or indentations
- *Flat* can describe a lesion, an area of interest, or an entire specimen.

Tissues commonly affected
Any

Common etiology
N/A

Sample gross description
"Present on the skin surface is a centrally located, dark-tan, irregular, **flat** lesion measuring . . . "

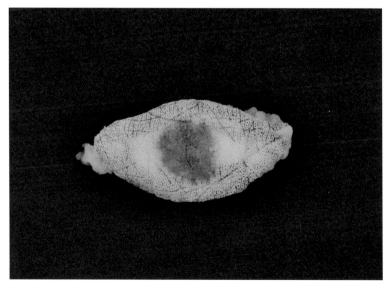

A flat lesion in the central part of a skin excision

Flecked

Gross appearance and identification
Small markings, streaks, or speckles, usually on serosal or mucosal surfaces
- Flecks on surfaces can indicate an underlying disease process.

Tissues commonly affected
Gallbladder

Common etiology
Cholesterolosis

Sample gross description
"The mucosa is yellow-**flecked** . . . "

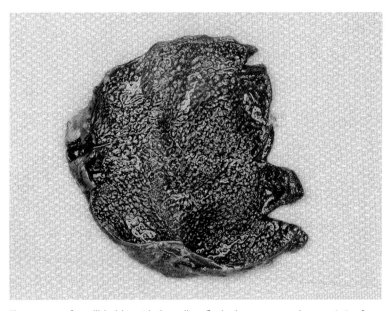

The mucosa of a gallbladder with the yellow-flecked appearance characteristic of cholesterolosis

Fleshy

Gross appearance and identification

A homogeneous, often tan or light-tan cut surface consisting of, or resembling, flesh

- Often, this cut surface involves lymph nodes or soft tissues that are associated with lymphoma and are likely encapsulated.

Tissues commonly affected

Lymph nodes, any soft tissue

Common etiology

Lymphoma, sarcoma, carcinoid, gastrointestinal stromal tumor (GIST)

Sample gross description

"The specimen is bivalved to reveal a single, well-circumscribed lesion with a homogeneous, pink-tan, **fleshy** cut surface."

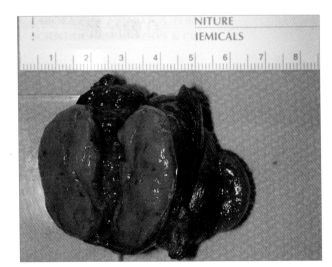

A thyroid that has been bisected to exhibit a solitary lesion with a fleshy cut surface

Fluid-filled

Gross appearance and identification

A structure, usually a cyst, that contains fluid

- Cysts and cavities often contain various types of fluid and are thus referred to as "fluid-filled."
- *Fluid-filled* is usually followed by another descriptive term, such as *cyst* or *cavity*, to explain the full meaning of the term.

Tissues commonly affected

Cysts, cavities, lungs

Common etiology

Serous or mucinous cystadenoma, blisters, pulmonary edema

Sample gross description

"The specimen is bisected to reveal a **fluid-filled** cystic mass, with a mostly smooth inner lining, and a focal red-and-yellow solid lesion."

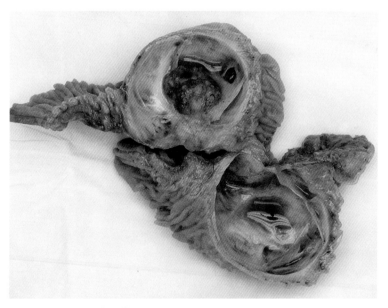

A large bowel with a fluid-filled submucosal cystic lesion

Focal

Gross appearance and identification
A localized area of interest
- In gross pathology, there are often specific areas of interest that are located within normal or abnormal areas.

Tissues commonly affected
Any

Common etiology
N/A

Sample gross description
"The cut surface shows a light-tan, nodular, cut surface with a **focal** area of possible fat necrosis measuring . . . "

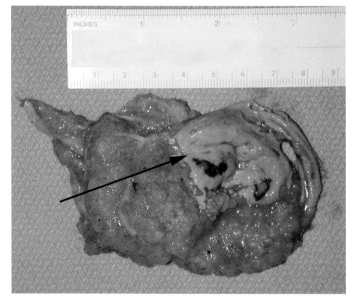

A focal area of fat necrosis (arrow) in the upper quadrant of the specimen

Fractured

Gross appearance and identification
Broken or ruptured bone or other firm tissue
  • *Fractured* mostly applies to bone or boney specimens, but
    can also apply to other firm tissues, such as gallstones.

Tissues commonly affected
Bones, cartilage

Common etiology
Trauma or bone tumors (including metastatic tumors)

Sample gross description
"The specimen consists of multiple portions of **fractured** bone,
skin, and grossly identifiable toes with attached nails . . . "

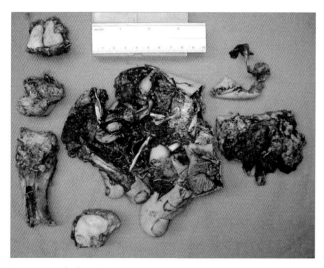

The bones of a foot that have been fractured as a result of trauma

Friable

Gross appearance and identification
Tissue that is easily broken into small fragments or reduced to powder
- In general, friable tissue in the pathology lab can be attributed to tissue necrosis or to the drying out of tissue.

Tissues commonly affected
Any

Common etiology
Tissue necrosis, drying out of tissue, gallstones

Sample gross description
"The specimen consists of multiple **friable**, deeply congested, and dark-tan portions of tissue measuring in aggregate . . . "

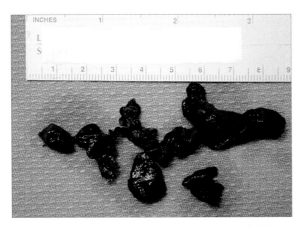

Hemorrhagic tissue fragments that show this tissue is friable (it easily falls apart during handling)

Fungating

Gross appearance and identification
A well-defined, ulcerating, and necrotic lesion
- A fungating lesion is often accompanied with a foul odor.
- It is typically seen in advanced-stage disease.

Tissues commonly affected
Skin

Common etiology
Breast cancer; skin cancers, including melanoma and squamous cell carcinoma

Sample gross description
"Present on the skin surface is a well-circumscribed, ulcerated, **fungating** lesion measuring . . . "

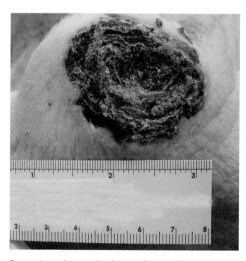

Fungating, ulcerated, advanced-stage skin cancer

Gangrenous

Gross appearance and identification
Darkened and/or mummified tissue
- The skin surface can be partially or entirely sloughed off.
- Diseased areas are often sharply demarcated from normal-appearing areas.
- Gangrenous tissue is essentially the death and decay of body tissue, often occurring in a limb, caused by insufficient blood supply and usually following injury or disease.

Tissues commonly affected
Extremities

Common etiology
Diabetes, infection, injury

Sample gross description
"The distal and plantar surface of the foot has a necrotic and **gangrenous** appearance."

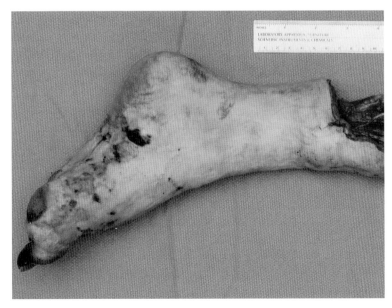

A below-knee amputation with extensive gangrene and necrosis at the distal aspect, due to a lack of vascular function as a result of diabetes

Gaseous

Gross appearance and identification
A lesion or gross appearance that is full of, or contains, gas
- In gross pathology, gas is often identified in the GI tract where free air can be trapped easily.
- Gas can also occur in other areas of the body due to localized trauma, infections, necrosis, or bacterial infections.

Tissues commonly affected
Stomach, intestines, pleura, lungs

Common etiology
Inflammatory bowel disease (IBD), pneumothorax, celiac disease, malabsorption, trauma

Sample gross description
"The pericardial sac has diffuse cystic, **gaseous** cavities and measures in aggregate . . . "

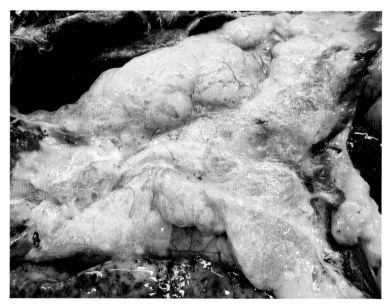

A pericardial sac that appears to have trapped gas as a result of traumatic chest compressions

Granulated

Gross appearance and identification
A surface or lining of a specimen with small grains or granules
- This is a common and grossly unremarkable appearance for many specimens.
- In gross pathology, it is important to note the appearance even if it is unremarkable, or clinically insignificant.

Tissues commonly affected
Appendix, bowel, peritoneal surfaces, other abdominal organs

Common etiology
Appendicitis, bowel perforation, peritonitis

Sample gross description
"The mucosa of the specimen appears mostly tan and **granulated** . . . "

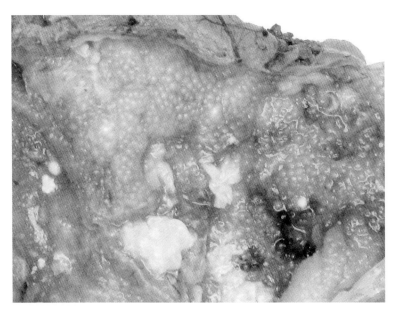

The mucosal surface of a colon that appears granular and absent of normal mucosal folds

Gritty

Gross appearance and identification
Composed of, or covered with, particles resembling grit in texture or consistency
- Calcifications may be present in gritty specimens, which may make them difficult to cut.
- The tissue is firm on palpation.

Tissues commonly affected
Soft tissues, cartilage

Common etiology
Calciphylaxis, ductal carcinoma in situ, pilomatrixoma

Sample gross description
"The specimen is serially sectioned to reveal a yellow/white, diffuse, heterogenous, speckled, **gritty** cut surface."

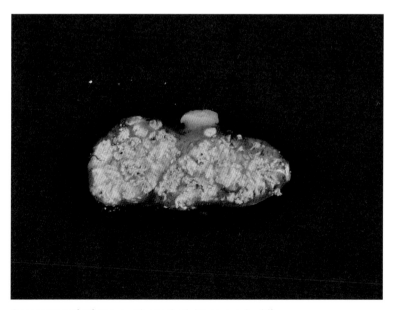

Cross section of soft tissue with attached skin to reveal a diffuse, gritty appearance

Hairy

Gross appearance and identification
Specimens that contain hair or material of similar appearance
- Most skin specimens contain various amounts of hair and can be referred to as *hair-bearing*.

Tissues commonly affected
Skin, ovaries, spine, periorbital region

Common etiology
Dermoid cysts (cystic teratoma)

Sample gross description
"The specimen is sectioned to reveal a cystic cavity filled with **hairy** and scant, tan, soft material."

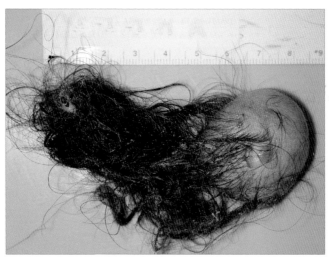

A dermoid cyst that has been opened to reveal a large amount of hair (common in this pathologic abnormality)

Hemorrhagic

Gross appearance and identification
Excessive aggregates of blood as a result of profuse bleeding
- Blood can accumulate anywhere, such as between tissue layers, on surfaces, or in lumens.
- Excessive accumulation of blood usually indicates an underlying pathologic process.

Tissues commonly affected
Any

Common etiology
Trauma, ulcerated lesions, varices

Sample gross description
"The lumen is dilated, and contains **hemorrhagic** material that measures in aggregate . . . "

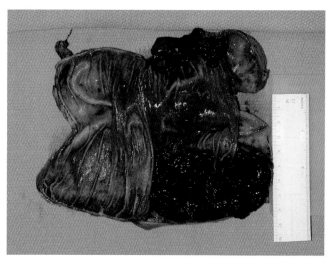

A mass of hemorrhage that has accumulated in the lumen of a bowel, the result of bleeding from trauma

Heterogeneous

Gross appearance and identification
Tissue or specimens that consist of dissimilar elements or parts
  • *Heterogeneous* is the exact opposite of *homogeneous.*

Tissues commonly affected
Any

Common etiology
Malignant tumors

Sample gross description
"The cut surface reveals a well-circumscribed, encapsulated mass with a **heterogeneous** appearance."

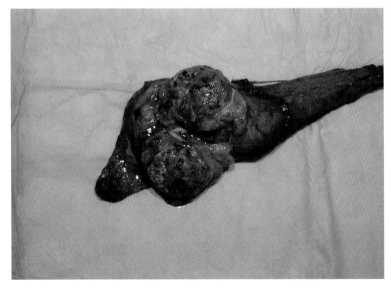

A testicle that has been bisected to reveal a malignant tumor with a heterogeneous appearance

Homogeneous

Gross appearance and identification
Tissue or specimens with an undifferentiated or uniform appearance
- In gross pathology, *homogeneous* can apply to a particular lesion or to an entire specimen.

Tissues commonly affected
Any

Common etiology
Lipoma, sarcoma, lymphoma

Sample gross description
"The specimen is bisected to reveal a well-circumscribed, yellow, **homogeneous** lesion measuring . . . "

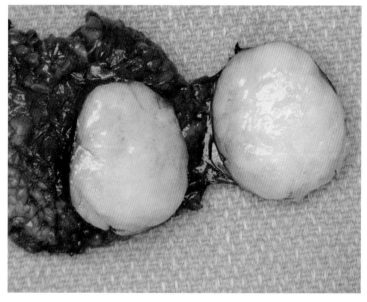

The cut surface of a lesion showing homogeneous color and consistency

Honeycomb

Gross appearance and identification
A lesion characterized by multiple similar or variably sized hexagonal (or similar) cystic spaces or structures

Tissues commonly affected
Lung, soft tissue, bone

Common etiology
Widespread fibrosis, pneumonia (lung), cystic degeneration

Sample gross description
"The specimen is longitudinally sectioned to reveal a cut surface of which half is dense, firm, gray-tan, and homogenous, and half is hemorrhagic and multicystic with a **honeycomb** appearance."

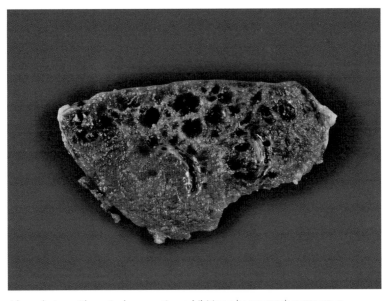

A bone lesion with cystic degeneration exhibiting a honeycomb appearance

Ill-defined

Gross appearance and identification

A lesion or area of interest that does not have a defined border

- Malignant lesions can present as ill-defined, as they metastasize locally and infiltrate surrounding tissue.

Tissues commonly affected

Any

Common etiology

Invasive ductal carcinoma, pulmonary nodules, ill-defined hypoechoic nodule

Sample gross description

"The specimen is sectioned to reveal a firm, **ill-defined** fibrous lesion measuring . . . "

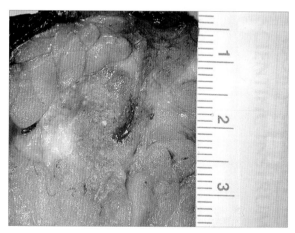

An ill-defined, invasive breast tumor that has infiltrated the surrounding parenchyma

Incised

Gross appearance and identification
A clean cut, as with a surgical knife

- Some specimens received in the pathology lab have been surgically removed because of traumatic incisions that have compromised the function of the organ, such as stab wounds.
- In many cases, surgeons incise specimens after removal to view lesions or organs before sending them to the pathology lab.

Tissues commonly affected
Any

Common etiology
Trauma, iatrogenic defect

Sample gross description
"There is a lateral **incision** present on the skin surface, located between the suture lines, measuring . . . "

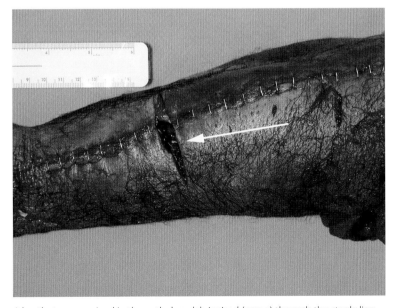

A leg that was received in the pathology lab incised (arrow) through the staple line

Indrawn

Gross appearance and identification
An area of interest that has been pulled inward in comparison to surrounding tissue
- An indrawn appearance is usually due to a pathologic process in the underlying tissue.

Tissues commonly affected
Skin, GI tract

Common etiology
Inflammatory bowel disease

Sample gross description
"Present on the large bowel mucosa is a linear, **indrawn** lesion measuring . . . "

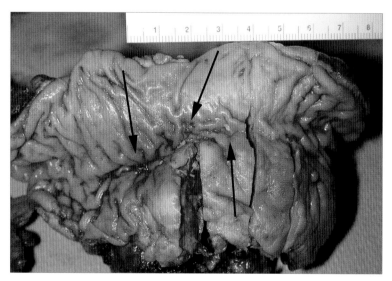

The mucosa of a large bowel with a large linear ulceration (arrows) that has caused the bowel to become indrawn for most of its length

Infarct

Gross appearance and identification
A dark-tan-to-black area of necrosis
- Infarcts can be localized to specific areas or can affect an entire organ.
- An infarct is tissue that undergoes necrosis as a result of obstruction of local blood supply, as by a thrombus or embolus.

Tissues commonly affected
Any

Common etiology
Myocardial infarction

Sample gross description
"The cut surface reveals a well-circumscribed, encapsulated lesion with lobular features and focal areas of **infarct**."

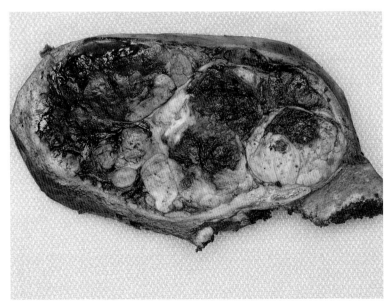

An infarct that has occurred in the blood supply to a liver tumor, causing areas of necrosis

Infiltrated

Gross appearance and identification
A permeation of a suspected malignant process or substance into adjacent and surrounding tissues
- *Infiltrated* is mostly used to describe the extent of a malignant neoplasm and its gross invasion through tissue layers.

Tissues commonly affected
Any

Common etiology
Malignant tumors

Sample gross description
"The cut surface shows gross **infiltration** of the tumor into the surrounding parenchyma . . . "

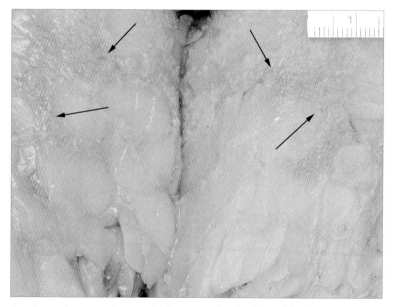

A malignant breast carcinoma, which originated in the ducts of the breast, that has grossly infiltrated (arrows) the surrounding breast parenchyma

Intact

Gross appearance and identification
Uncompromised surfaces or membranes
- *Intact* grossly refers to the appearance of specimens when they arrive at the pathology lab.
- Nonintact specimens have a compromised appearance as a result of a surgery or a pathologic process.

Tissues commonly affected
All

Common etiology
N/A

Sample gross description
"The specimen consists of an **intact** gallbladder measuring . . . "

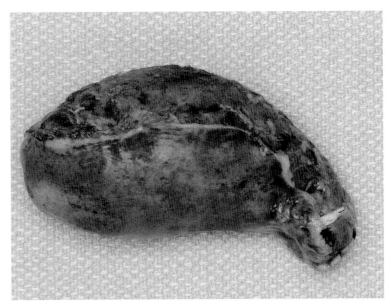

A gallbladder that is intact in appearance because the serosal surface is not compromised

Intermixed

Gross appearance and identification
Tissue that has broken down into small fragments, and been
removed manually or through suction, with accompanying
blood, soft tissue, or bone

Tissues commonly affected
Bone, blood clots, mucous, soft tissue

Common etiology
Curettage, debridement

Sample gross description
"The specimen consists of multiple gray-white bone fragments
intermixed with blood clot and measuring in aggregate…"

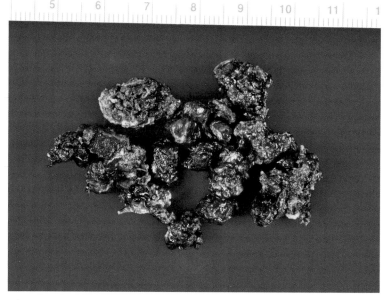

A bone curettage specimen intermixed with blood clot (it would be difficult to
separate the bone fragments from the blood clot in this case)

Intracavitary

Gross appearance and identification
A lesion or area of interest that is located within an organ or body cavity

- *Intracavitary* can also refer to the center of a lesion that is necrotic due to infection (i.e., an abscess) or cancer (tumor necrosis).

Tissues commonly affected
Any

Common etiology
Infections, tumors

Sample gross description
"The specimen is bivalved to reveal a white-whorled, well-circumscribed **intracavitary** mass measuring . . . "

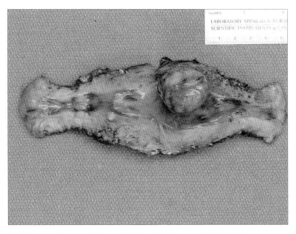

An intracavitary endometrial fibroid (located within the endometrial cavity of the uterus)

Intraluminal

Gross appearance and identification
A lesion or process that occurs within the lumen of a specimen
- Pathologic processes can develop on luminal walls, causing outgrowths into luminal spaces.

Tissues commonly affected
Any luminal structure including GI tract, fallopian tubes, vessels

Common etiology
Tumors, ectopic pregnancy

Sample gross description
"The lumen is cross sectioned to reveal a well-circumscribed, tan, homogeneous **intraluminal** mass measuring . . . "

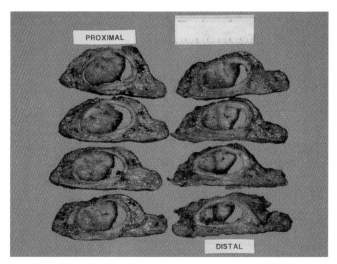

Cross sections of colon that show a malignant polyp, which arises from the mucosal lining, protruding into the lumen and causing an obstruction

Invasive

Gross appearance and identification
A disease or condition that has spread, especially a malignant cancer that has spread into healthy tissue

- *Invade* or *invasive* are used to describe the gross extent of a pathologic process.

Tissues commonly affected
Any

Common etiology
Malignant tumors

Sample gross description
"The tumor appears to **invade** through the muscle layers and wall of the large intestine into the surrounding pericolic fat."

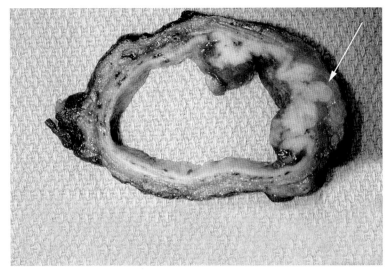

A malignant neoplasm, which originated as a mucosal lesion and has invaded (arrow) the mucosa, muscle layers, wall of the large intestine, and the surrounding pericolic fat

Inverted

Gross appearance and identification
A lesion or specific gross appearance that has been reversed in position, direction, or order

Tissues commonly affected
Breast

Common etiology
Malignant tumor

Sample gross description
"The nipple is eccentrically located and **inverted**, and measures . . . "

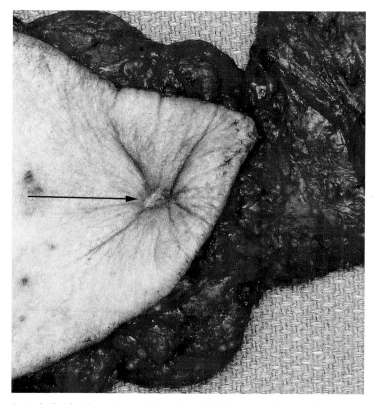

A nipple that has been inverted (arrow) probably because of an underlying malignant tumor

Irregular

Gross appearance and identification
Specimens and lesions that do not have a definitive, classical appearance

Tissues commonly affected
Any

Common etiology
N/A

Sample gross description
"The specimen consists of an **irregular** portion of bowel mucosa measuring . . . "

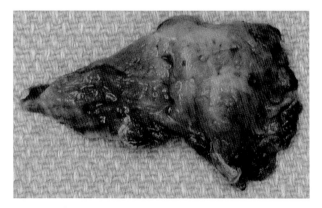

A portion of bowel mucosa that has an overall irregular shape

Ischemic

Gross appearance and identification
A lesion or area of interest that is dark-tan, deeply congested, and/or necrotic
  • Ischemia is inadequate blood supply to a part of the body, caused by partial or total blockage of an artery.

Tissues commonly affected
GI tract, legs, kidneys, feet, heart

Common etiology
Coronary artery disease, stroke, angina, transient ischemic attack (TIA)

Sample gross description
"The specimen consists of a segmental resection of small bowel, which has an overall **ischemic** appearance, and measures . . . "

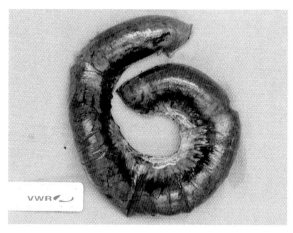

A segment of ischemic small bowel, which has become nonfunctional due to a reduced blood supply

Laceration

Gross appearance and identification
A cut or wound that looks jagged
- In gross pathology, lacerations are usually present in cases involving trauma.

Tissues commonly affected
Any

Common etiology
Trauma

Sample gross description
"The splenectomy specimen shows multiple linear **lacerations** as a result of trauma."

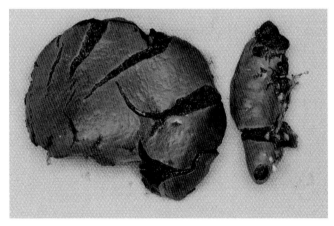

A below-knee amputation as a result of trauma, with a laceration that appears to have been done postsurgically

Lamellate (lamellar)

Gross appearance and identification
An organ, process, or structure with thin layers, plates or scales

Tissues commonly affected
Bone (haversian canals), placentae, teeth, soft tissues

Common etiology
Thrombi (formed by gradual clotting of blood in successive layers, or laminations: lighter layers are fibrin, darker layers are red blood cells)

Sample gross description
"The specimen is serially sectioned to reveal a single, well-circumscribed, ovoid mass with a hemorrhagic, tan, **lamellate** cut surface measuring . . . "

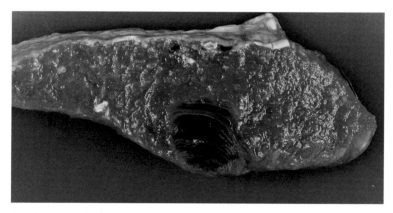

A well-circumscribed intervillous thrombus in a parenchyma of the placenta exhibiting lamellate features

Linear

Gross appearance and identification
A line, or an appearance resembling a line
- In pathology, a linear appearance is most commonly associated with scarring from a previous surgery or underlying disease process.

Tissues commonly affected
Skin, GI tract

Common etiology
Scarring from previous surgery, inflammatory bowel disease

Sample gross description
"Present on the skin surface is a centrally located, well-healed **linear** scar measuring . . . "

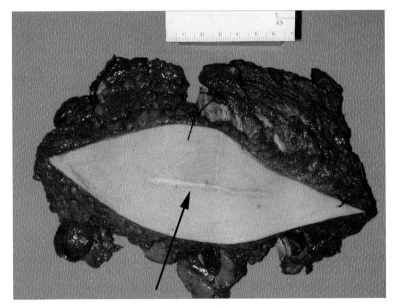

Skin with a centrally located linear scar (arrow) from a previous surgery

Lobulated

Gross appearance and identification
Multiple, rounded, often homogeneous-appearing lobules
- *Lobulated* is most often used to refer to fatty tissue specimens.
- It can be used to describe normal-appearing tissue, but can refer to lipomatous tumors.

Tissues commonly affected
Subcutaneous tissue, breast

Common etiology
Lipoma, liposarcoma

Sample gross description
"The specimen is bisected to reveal a homogeneous, yellow, **lobulated** cut surface."

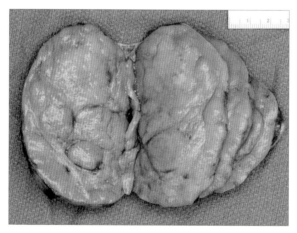

A lipoma with a classic yellow, lobulated appearance

Loculated

Gross appearance and identification
Multiple small cavities contained within a larger structure
- Loculated lesions can occur in most parts of the body, but are most common in the lungs and ovaries.
- They may indicate an underlying disease process.

Tissues commonly affected
Lungs, ovaries

Common etiology
Loculated empyema, loculated pleural effusion, ovarian cysts

Sample gross description
"The specimen is opened to reveal a **loculated** cyst, with loculi that range in size from . . . "

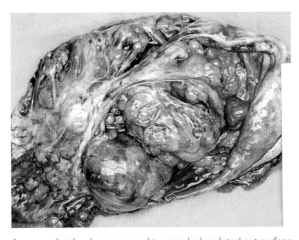

An ovary that has been opened to reveal a loculated cut surface

Macronodular

Gross appearance and identification
A lesion or area of interest characterized by large nodules
(> 5 mm in diameter)

- In gross pathology, *macronodular* is usually reserved for
larger skin or mucosal lesions.

Tissues commonly affected
Skin, mucosal surfaces

Common etiology
Candidiasis, erythematous macronodular skin lesions, rash

Sample gross description
"Present on the skin surface are multiple, unevenly distributed
macronodular lesions ranging in size from . . . "

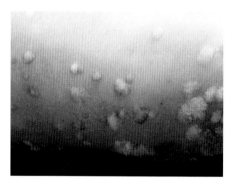

A skin lesion exhibiting a typical large, or
macronodular, appearance

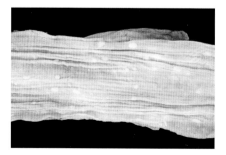

Small bowel mucosa with multiple
macronodular lesions

Macule

Gross appearance and identification
A small, flat, colored spot
- *Macule* is usually understood to refer to a spot on a mucosal surface or on the skin.

Tissues commonly affected
Skin, mucosal surfaces

Common etiology
Freckles, rash

Sample gross description
"Present on the skin surface is a centrally located, well-defined oval **macule** measuring . . . "

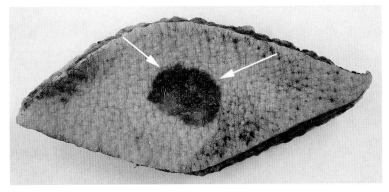

A dark-tan, centrally located macule (arrows) that is a benign melanocytic lesion

Mammillated

Gross appearance and identification
A lesion or area of interest that is studded with, or possesses, nipple-like projections or protuberances
  • Mammillated appearance does not indicate benign or malignant etiology.

Tissues commonly affected
Any, but most common on skin, bone, and mucosal surfaces

Common etiology
Skin tags, exostosis

Sample gross description
"Present on the chest wall are 2 **mammillated** lesions measuring . . . "

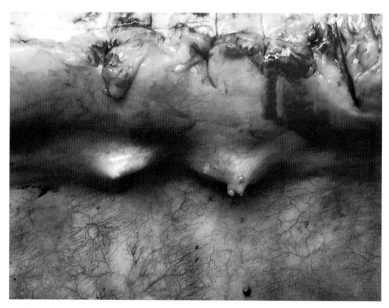

Two boney protuberances, or mammillated lesions, from a chest cavity

Miliary

Gross appearance and identification
An area of interest characterized by lesions resembling small seeds

- *Miliary* comes from *millet*, which is a grain with small seeds.
- The "millet seeds" correspond to granulomas and can also be seen in disseminated histoplasmosis and cytomegalovirus (CMV) pneumonitis.

Tissues commonly affected
Skin, but can affect any organ system

Common etiology
Miliary tuberculosis

Sample gross description
"The specimen is sectioned to reveal a **miliary** cut surface."

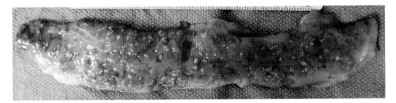

A pancreas with a classic millet-seed or miliary appearance on its cut surface

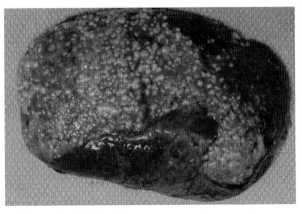

A spleen with a classic miliary appearance on its cut surface

Mottled

Gross appearance and identification
Tissue with spots or blotches of different shades or colors
- Mottling results from cutaneous ischemia or changes in vascular supply.

Tissues commonly affected
Skin

Common etiology
Livedo reticularis, herpes zoster infections

Sample gross description
"The specimen is bivalved to reveal multiple dark-red lesions distributed in a **mottled** pattern."

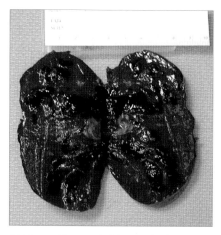

A kidney with a mottled, hemorrhagic appearance

Mucinous

Gross appearance and identification
Aggregates of mucous
- In some parts of the body, such as the stomach, the production of mucous is normal. However, some pathologic processes can exhibit an overproduction of mucous.

Tissues commonly affected
Breast, appendix, ovaries

Common etiology
Pseudomyxoma peritonei, mucinous cyst adenoma, mucinous cyst adenocarcinoma, mucinous breast lesions

Sample gross description
"The specimen is opened to reveal a cystic cavity that is filled with **mucinous** material."

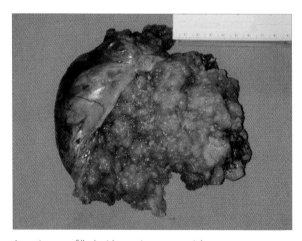

A cystic ovary filled with mucinous material

Multicystic

Gross appearance and identification
Multiple saclike structures or cysts
 • This gross appearance is also referred to as *polycystic*.

Tissues commonly affected
Ovaries, kidneys

Common etiology
Polycystic kidney disease, polycystic ovary

Sample gross description
"The specimen consists of a **multicystic**, ovoid mass measuring . . . "

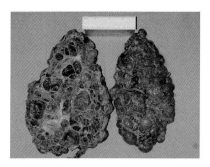

A kidney that has been bisected to reveal a multicystic cut surface, which is characteristic of polycystic kidney disease

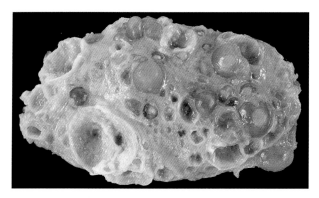

A cross section of an ovary with a multicystic appearance

Multifaceted

Gross appearance and identification
Grossly appears as having many facets or aspects

Tissues commonly affected
Gallbladder

Common etiology
Cholelithiasis

Sample gross description
"The lumen contains multiple brown **multifaceted** calculi ranging in size from . . . "

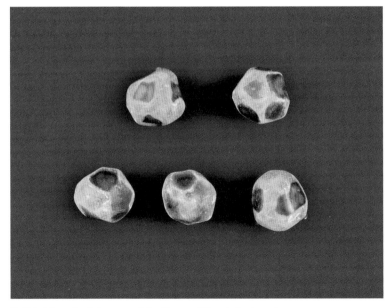

Gallbladder calculi that are solid, with a multifaceted external appearance

Multifocal

Gross appearance and identification

A lesion, abnormality, or area of interest that has multiple points of origin

- *Multifocal* is especially useful as a way to describe multiple lesions without having to describe each lesion individually.

Tissues commonly affected

Colon, breast, thyroid

Common etiology

Multifocal breast cancer, metastatic lesions

Sample gross description

"The mucosa of the large intestine contains multiple **multifocal** lobulated lesions ranging in size from . . . "

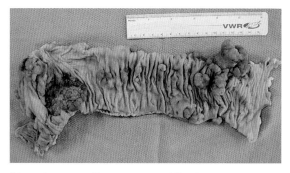

A bowel mucosa with numerous multifocal tumors

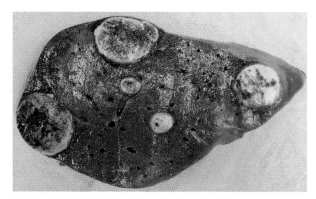

Four multifocal tumors on the cut surface of a liver

Multilobular

Gross appearance and identification
A lesion or area of interest that contains many lobules
- *Multilobular* is often used to describe the appearance of soft-tissue tumors and bone tumors.

Tissues commonly affected
Bone, soft tissues

Common etiology
Multilobular osteomas and chondromas; sarcomas; lipomas

Sample gross description
"The specimen is sectioned to reveal a heterogeneous, **multilobular** cut surface."

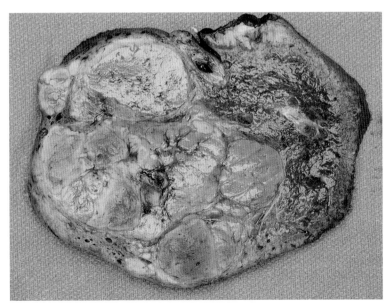

The cut surface of a multilobulated soft-tissue sarcoma

Multiparous

Gross appearance and identification
A slit-like opening in the cervical os

Tissues commonly affected
Cervix

Common etiology
Usually evidence of having given birth

Sample gross description
"The cervical os appears **multiparous** and measures . . . "

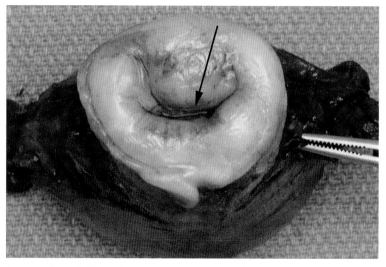

A cervix with a slit-like, multiparous appearance (arrow)

Mummified

Gross appearance and identification
Dark-tan-to-black, necrotic, firm tissue
- Tissues that have a mummified appearance often have a compromised blood supply, which causes the affected tissue to shrivel and dry up.

Tissues commonly affected
Extremities

Common etiology
Peripheral vascular disease, diabetes

Sample gross description
"The distal foot appears to be gangrenous and the digits are **mummified**."

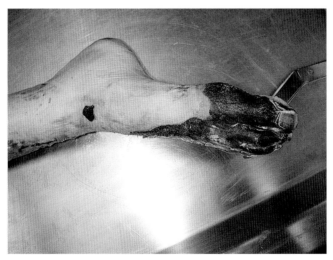

Mummification in the right foot of a patient whose diabetes has occluded the foot's vascular supply

Necrotic

Gross appearance and identification
Tan or dark-tan tissue that easily breaks apart (friable)
- *Necrosis* refers to the death of cells or tissues from injury or disease, especially in a localized area of the body.

Tissues commonly affected
Any

Common etiology
Ischemia, trauma

Sample gross description
"The cut surface appears yellow/brown and **necrotic**."

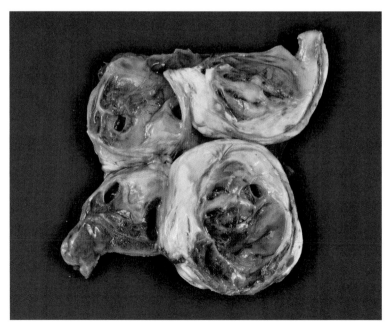

Soft tissue exhibiting extensive tissue necrosis

Nodular

Gross appearance and identification
Grossly appears as a specimen or area of interest having or resembling nodules.

Tissues commonly affected
Any

Common etiology
Nodular dermatofibrosis, nodular hyperplasia, nodular thyroid hyperplasia

Sample gross description
"Contained within the lumen are 2 yellow, ovoid calculi with a **nodular** appearance measuring . . . "

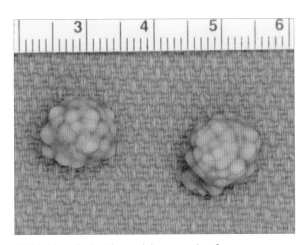

Gallbladder calculi with a nodular external surface

Nodule

Gross appearance and identification
A small (up to 1 cm in diameter) bump, node, swelling, or protuberance

- Nodules are characterized by being elevated and up to 1 cm in size.

Tissues commonly affected
Any

Common etiology
Cutaneous nodule, renal nodule, rheumatoid nodule, satellite nodule, Sister Mary Joseph nodule, solitary thyroid nodule

Sample gross description
"Present on the serosal surface is a focal light-tan **nodule** measuring . . . "

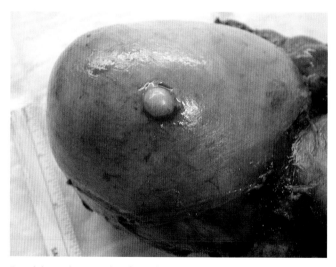

A nodule on the serosal surface of the uterine fundus

Nonintact

Gross appearance and identification
A defect in a specimen that alters its natural appearance
* Specimens can be altered by a pathologic process or as a result of a surgical procedure.

Tissues commonly affected
Any

Common Causes
Trauma, perforations

Sample gross description
"The surface of the specimen appears **nonintact,** exposing the inner contents."

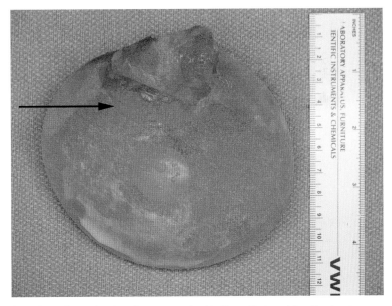

A nonintact breast implant that was received in the pathology lab with a tearing defect (arrow) in the capsule

Nulliparous

Gross appearance and identification
A pinhole opening of the cervical os

Tissues commonly affected
Cervix

Common etiology
Women who have not given birth present with a nulliparous os.

Sample gross description
"The cervical os is **nulliparous** and measures . . . "

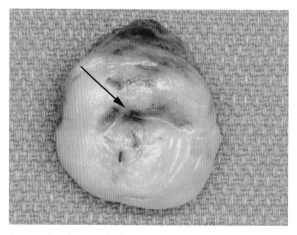

A cervical os that is pinhole or nulliparous in appearance
(arrow)

Obstructed

Gross appearance and identification

A luminal structure that has been blocked, or filled with obstacles or an obstacle

Tissues commonly affected

Luminal structures such as vessels, GI tract, fallopian tube, biliary tree

Common etiology

Myocardial infarction, bowel obstruction, cholecystitis, ectopic pregnancy

- Obstructions can prevent normal flow or transit in luminal structures, causing impairment and inability of an organ system to operate.
- In vessels, obstructions can cause ischemia, acute tissue damage, and possibly death if occurring in the heart or brain.

Sample gross description

"The hepatic duct is dilated and **obstructed** by a dark-tan calculus measuring . . . "

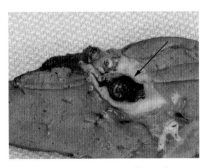

A duct in the liver obstructed by gallstones

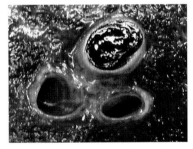

An obstructed vessel next to 2 patent vessels

Oval

Gross appearance and identification
An overall specimen shape that is oval
- *Oval* refers to a 2-dimensional appearance.

Tissues commonly affected
Any

Common etiology
N/A

Sample gross description
"The specimen consists of an **oval** portion of skin with underlying subcutaneous tissue measuring . . . "

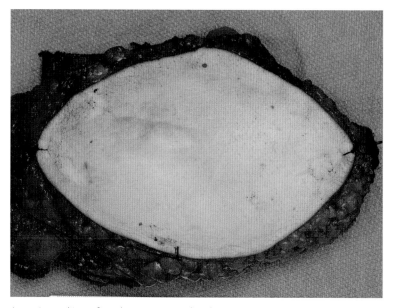

A specimen skin surface that appears oval in shape

Ovoid

Gross appearance and identification
Specimens or lesions with an overall egg shape
- Note that *ovoid* is a 3-dimensional description, whereas *oval* is a 2-dimensional description.

Tissues commonly affected
Ovaries, cysts

Common etiology
Conditions affecting the ovaries; carcinomas; cyst adenomas

Sample gross description
"The specimen consists of an **ovoid**, cystic mass measuring . . . "

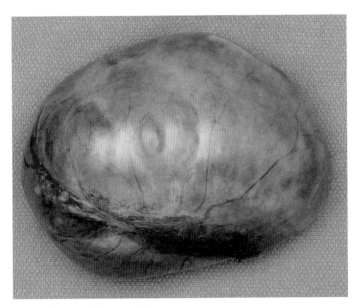

An ovarian cyst with an ovoid shape

Papillary

Gross appearance and identification
A lesion or area of interest that resembles a papilla
- Papillary lesions may indicate a malignant or premalignant process.

Tissues commonly affected
Ovary, thyroid

Common etiology
Papillary thyroid carcinoma, borderline ovarian tumors

Sample gross description
"The cut surface reveals a solid-cystic lesion containing opaque fluid with **papillary** features."

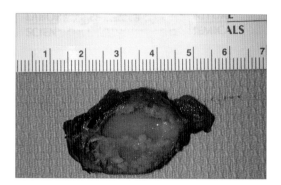

A cross section of thyroid showing a cyst that contains a papillary lesion and fluid

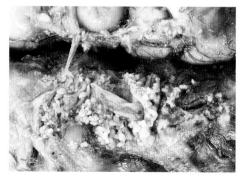

A papillary lesion forming on the surface of the brain

Papillate

Gross appearance and identification

Covered by papillae or nipple-like prominences

- Papillae are most commonly seen on the tongue surface, but can be observed in other areas, most often mucosal surfaces.

Tissues commonly affected

Tongue, other mucosal surfaces, skin

Common etiology

Papillary hyperplasia

Sample gross description

"The tongue appears **papillate** and normal . . . "

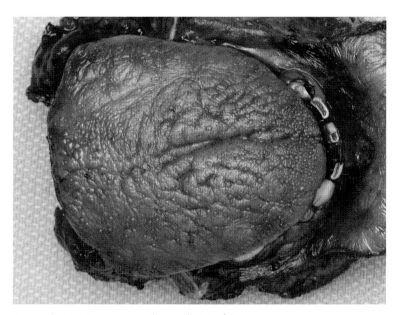

A normal-appearing tongue with a papillate surface

Papule

Gross appearance and identification
A small (> 1 cm in diameter), circumscribed, superficial, solid, elevated lesion

- Papules most commonly occur on skin and mucous membranes, but can occur on other parts of the body.
- Most papules are benign.

Tissues commonly affected
Skin, mucous membranes

Common etiology
Pimples, syphilis, hyperplastic colon polyps

Sample gross description
"The mucosa of the large bowel has 2 focal **papules**, which measure . . . "

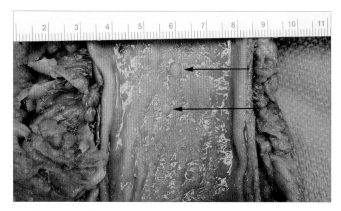

Two distinct papules (arrows) on the mucosal surface of a bowel

Patent

Gross appearance and identification
An open or unobstructed luminal structure
- Luminal structures include ducts, lumens, and vessels.
- Many diseases can affect the patency of luminal structures including inflammation, tumors, and obstructions.

Tissues commonly affected
Ducts, lumens and vessels

Common etiology
N/A

Sample gross description
"The bile duct is opened to reveal that it is slightly dilated and **patent**."

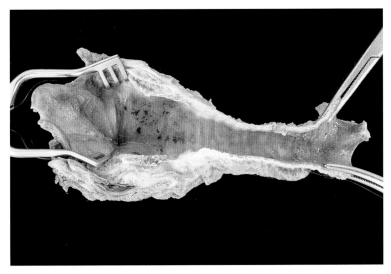

An opened and patent trachea

Peau d'orange

Gross appearance and identification
In a breast cancer mastectomy specimen, a swollen, dimpled, and pitted skin surface resembling the surface of an orange
- Peau d'orange arises from an underlying breast carcinoma in which there is both stromal infiltration and lymphatic obstruction with edema.

Tissues commonly affected
Skin surface of breast mastectomy specimens

Common etiology
Breast carcinoma, inflammatory breast cancer

Sample gross description
"The skin surface exhibits a **peau d' orange** appearance."

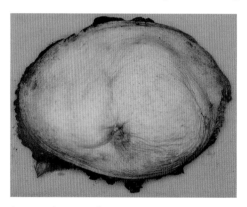

An extensive peau d'orange appearance

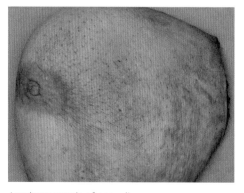

Another example of peau d'orange

Pedunculated polyp

Gross appearance and identification
A growth or mass with a thin stalk protruding from a mucous membrane
- Pedunculated polyps are usually an overgrowth of normal tissue, but can sometimes be true tumors (masses of new tissue separate from the supporting membrane).

Tissues commonly affected
Mucous membranes, skin, nose, ears, mouth, lungs, heart, stomach, intestines, urinary bladder, uterus, and cervix

Common etiology
Familial adenomatous polyposis, colon polyps, nasal polyps, skin tags

Sample gross description
"Present on the mucosal surface is a dark-tan **pedunculated polyp** measuring . . . "

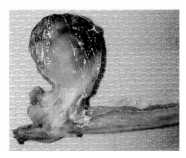

A pedunculated polyp arising from a large intestine mucosa

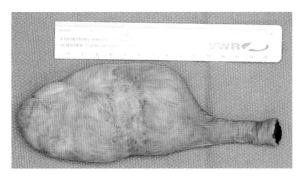

An excised pedunculated skin lesion with a classic thin stalk

Perforated

Gross appearance and identification

A hole or break in the containing walls or membranes of a structure or organ

- A perforation occurs when erosion, infection, or other factors create a weak area in an organ, and internal pressure causes a rupture.
- Perforations may also result from deep penetrating wounds caused by trauma.

Tissues commonly affected

Any

Common etiology

Trauma, inflammation, malignant tumors

Sample gross description

"The large bowel is opened to reveal a focal **perforation** measuring . . . "

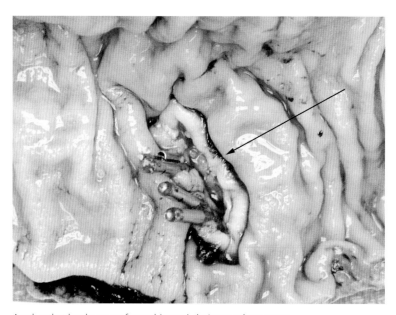

A colon that has been perforated (arrow) during a colonoscopy

Petechia

Gross appearance and identification
Small (< 3 mm in diameter) purplish spots on a body surface, such as the skin or a mucous membrane
- Petechia are caused by minor hemorrhages affecting capillaries.

Tissues commonly affected
Skin, mucous membranes

Common etiology
Trauma, meningococcemia, leukemia, and certain causes of thrombocytopenia

Sample gross description
"The mucosal surface has multiple dark-red **petechial** lesions distributed in an irregular pattern which measure . . . "

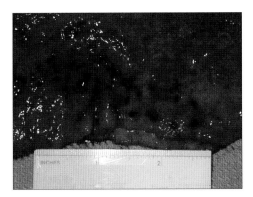
Petechia on the mucosal surface of the large intestine

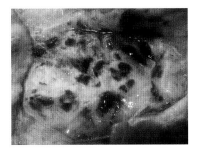
Petechia on the surface of the brain

Pigmented

Gross appearance and identification
Darkened lesions on light-colored background tissue
- *Pigmented* is most often used to describe skin spots that are brown or black.
- The lesions are usually moles and are colored as the result of a deposit of pigment.
- Pigmented lesions can have a variety of sizes, colors, and border shapes.

Tissues commonly affected
Skin, mucosal membranes

Common etiology
Melanoma, melanocytic nevus

Sample gross description
"Present on the skin surface is a centrally located dark-tan, **pigmented**, irregular, flat lesion measuring . . . "

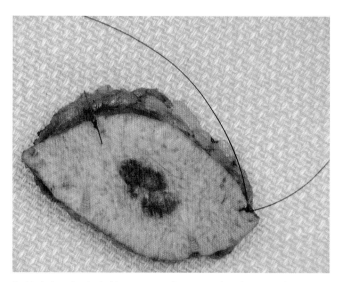

A skin lesion that is darkly pigmented compared to the normal surrounding skin

Plaque

Gross appearance and identification
A flat, often raised, patch on the skin or any other organ
- Plaque can come from abnormal mucous buildup or an accumulation of fatty deposits.

Tissues commonly affected
Vessels, skin, oral cavity, pleural cavity

Common etiology
Atherosclerosis, pseudomembranous colitis, psoriasis, mesothelioma

Sample gross description
"The mucosal surface has a diffuse pattern of adherent pale-yellow, rounded, **plaque** lesions which extend from the proximal resection margin to within . . . "

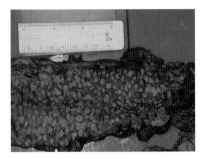

Multiple, diffuse plaques on the mucosal surface of the colon, which is typical in pseudomembranous colitis

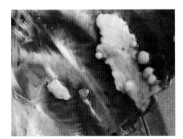

Mesothelioma, which presents here as a white adherent plaque on this chest wall

Protruding

Gross appearance and identification
Tissue or an abnormality that is pushed or thrust outward
- In gross pathology, *protruding* is mostly used to describe contents within an organ or specimen that are pushed outward from a luminal opening or defect.

Tissues commonly affected
Any

Common etiology
Endometrial cancer, rectal cancer

Sample gross description
"**Protruding** through the cervical os is a lobulated, yellow-tan and hemorrhagic, irregular mass measuring . . . "

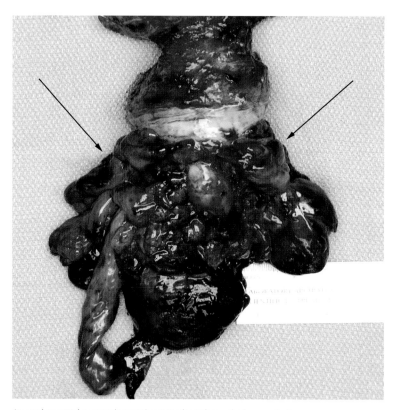

An endometrial cancer (arrows) protruding through the cervical os

Pseudocyst

Gross appearance and identification
An abnormal or dilated space or cavity resembling a cyst but not lined with epithelium
- Pseudocysts may contain gas or liquid, but they do not have a lining membrane.
- Pseudocysts are usually associated with benign pancreatic cysts.

Tissues commonly affected
Pancreas

Common etiology
Pseudocyst

Sample gross description
"The specimen is bivalved to reveal a possible **pseudocyst** filled with clear serous fluid measuring . . . "

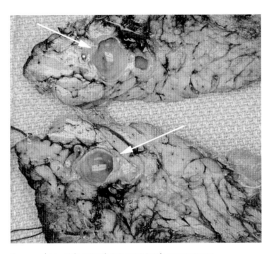

A pseudocyst (arrows) present in the pancreas

Pseudopolyp

Gross appearance and identification
A hypertrophied tab of mucous membrane resembling a polyp
- Pseudopolyps are typical of ulcerative colitis, but may be seen in other disease processes.

Tissues commonly affected
GI tract

Common etiology
IBD, bacterial dysentery, amebiasis due to *Entamoeba histolytica* and schistosomiasis

Sample gross description
"The large bowel mucosa has diffuse **pseudopolyps**, measuring from 0.2 cm to 0.5 cm, which extend from the proximal margin to . . . "

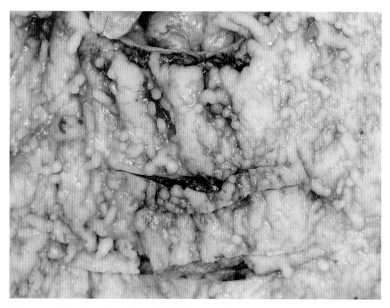

The mucosal surface of a colon with diffuse pseudopolyps due to IBD

Puckered

Gross appearance and identification
A focal area that exhibits a wrinkle, crease, or irregular fold
- *Puckering* often refers to a constriction or contraction of a surface due to an underlying disease process.

Tissues commonly affected
Any

Common etiology
Malignant lesions

Sample gross description
"The serosal surface appears mostly smooth except for a focal **puckered** lesion measuring . . . "

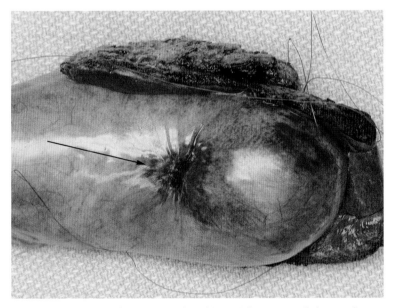

A gallbladder serosal surface that is puckered (arrow) due to an underlying malignant tumor

Pultaceous/sebaceous material

Gross appearance and identification
Soft, macerated, and often nearly fluid material
- *Pultaceous* is often used to describe the consistency of cystic contents that are soft and cheese-like.

Tissues commonly affected
Subcutaneous tissue, ovaries

Common etiology
Sebaceous cysts, dermoid cysts, epidermal inclusion cysts

Sample gross description
"The specimen is serially sectioned to reveal a cystic cavity, filled with yellow **pultaceous/sebaceous material**."

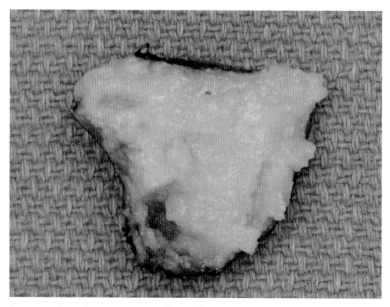

A cross section of a cyst showing yellow, pultaceous material within

Purulent/suppurating

Gross appearance and identification
A lesion or area of interest that forms pus

Tissues commonly affected
Any tissue in any part of the body

Common etiology
Result of the body's defensive reaction to foreign material
- Formation of pus is associated with an infectious process and contains digested tissue, white blood cells, and enzymes.

Sample gross description
"The specimen is incised to reveal a cystic cavity containing yellow **purulent/suppurative** material."

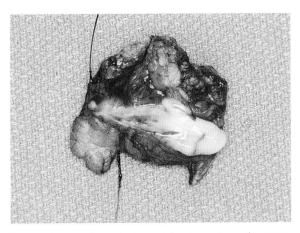

Purulent/suppurative material (pus) forming in tissue due to an underlying infection

Pus

Gross appearance and identification
A generally viscous, yellow-white fluid in infected tissue
- Pus consists of white blood cells, cellular debris, and necrotic tissue, which are usually products of inflammation.

Tissues commonly affected
Any

Common etiology
Abscesses, sores, infection

Sample gross description
"The specimen is incised to reveal a cystic cavity containing a plastic T-shaped intrauterine device surrounded by **pus**."

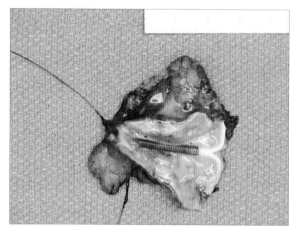

Soft tissue implanted with an intrauterine device (IUD), which has caused an infection producing pus

Pushing

Gross appearance and identification

A lesion or area of interest that appears to extend or push adjacent normal structures and may invade or infiltrate them

- Pushing lesions happen in all areas of the body, and can be malignant or benign.

Tissues commonly affected

Any

Common etiology

Malignant or benign neoplasms

Sample gross description

"The specimen is sectioned to reveal a heterogeneous neoplasm extending from the periosteum, **pushing** the muscle to give an outer, protruding appearance."

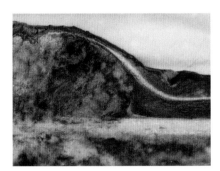

A bone lesion that appears to push the outer surface of a specimen, which gives the specimen a protruding appearance

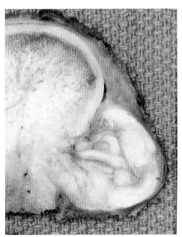

Another example of bone lesion pushing the outer surface of a specimen

Raised

Gross appearance and identification

A lesion or area of interest that is elevated above normal
surrounding tissue

- Raised lesions are most commonly associated with tumors,
  including localized swelling and edema.

Tissues commonly affected

Any

Common etiology

Tumors, edema, inflammation

Sample gross description

"Present on the anterior surface is a single, ovoid, **raised** lesion
with central ulceration and necrosis."

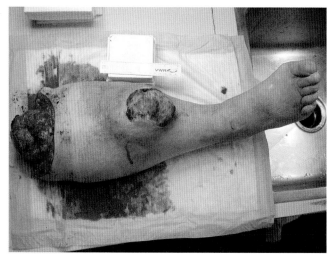

A sarcoma lesion that is ulcerated and raised above the normal-
appearing skin

Reniform

Gross appearance and identification
A specimen, lesion, or area of interest that has the shape or profile of a kidney

Tissues commonly affected
Kidney

Common etiology
N/A

Sample gross description
"The specimen consists of a left nephrectomy specimen, with classic **reniform** appearance, measuring . . . "

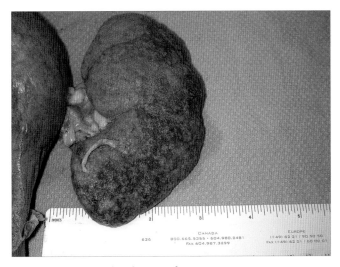

A kidney specimen with a classic reniform appearance

Roughened

Gross appearance and identification

A ragged, irregular, nonuniform area

- Roughened surfaces on specimens are tearing defects from pathologic processes, trauma, or difficulty in removing a specimen during surgery.

Tissues commonly affected

Any

Common etiology

Trauma

Sample gross description

"The serosal surface appears **roughened** with areas of adherent blood clot."

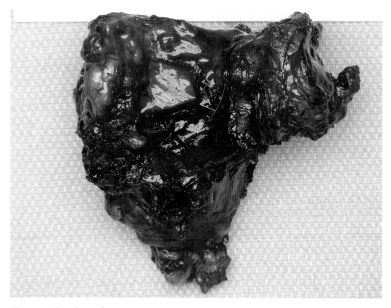

The serosal surface of a uterus that appears roughened due to the difficulty of a hysterectomy procedure

Ruptured

Gross appearance and identification
A tear or break in the continuity or configuration of tissue or an organ

- Ruptured specimens often display tearing or disruption of a membrane, or flattened tissue from being subjected to pressure.

Tissues commonly affected
Any

Common etiology
Appendicitis, ectopic pregnancy, trauma

Sample gross description
"The capsular surface appears **ruptured**, exposing the underlying parenchyma."

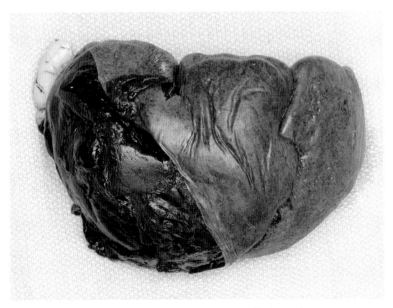

A spleen that was ruptured due to a traumatic motor vehicle accident

Scaled

Gross appearance and identification

A lesion or area of interest with thin flakes or compacted platelike structures, as of cornified epithelial cells on the body surface

- Scaling usually occurs due to a pathologic skin condition or as a result of dry skin.

Tissues commonly affected

Skin

Common etiology

Eczema, contact dermatitis, dry skin, actinic keratosis, psoriasis

Sample gross description

"The skin surface appears heterogeneous and roughened with areas of **scaling**."

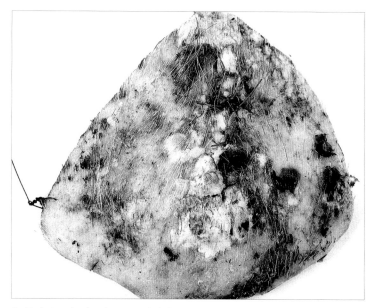

A skin lesion that has become slightly necrotic, with scaling features

Segmental

Gross appearance and identification

An excised part of an organ, gland, or other body part (due to surgery)

- Segmental resections can be performed for a variety of reasons, and remove only part of an organ. For example, a bowel resection removes part of the bowel, and leaves the remainder intact and functional.

Tissues commonly affected

Bowel, breast, thyroid, lung, liver

Common etiology

Malignant tumors, inflammatory bowel disease

Sample gross description

"The specimen consists of a **segmental** resection of terminal ileum, ileocecal valve, and proximal large intestine."

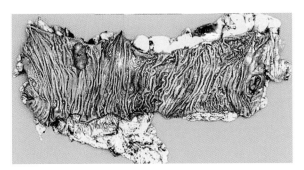

A segmental resection, so described because it involves only the distal small bowel (at right) and part of the proximal large colon

Septate

Gross appearance and identification
A lesion or area of interest that exhibits a separation or division by a septum or septa

- *Septate* usually applies to liver cysts, but can also apply to cysts in other parts of the body.

Tissues commonly affected
Uterus, liver, ovaries

Common etiology
Liver cysts, ovarian cysts

Sample gross description
"The specimen is sectioned to reveal multiple cystic cavities, separated by distinct **septate** borders, measuring from . . . "

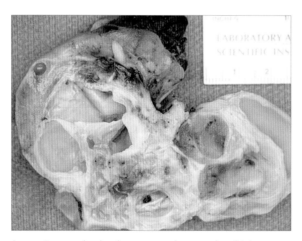

An ovarian cyst that has been opened to reveal multiple septate loculi

Serosal

Gross appearance and identification
A serous membrane, especially one that lines the pericardial, pleural, and peritoneal cavities, enclosing their contents
- *Serosal* applies to the specific surface that a grosser is referring to.

Tissues commonly affected
Pleura, pericardium, peritoneum, endocardium

Common etiology
N/A

Sample gross description
"The **serosal** surface appears smooth and unremarkable . . . "

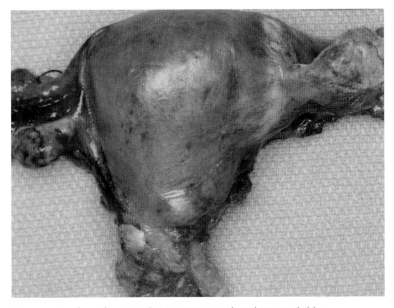

The serosal surface of a uterus that appears smooth and unremarkable

Serous fluid

Gross appearance and identification

Clear, pale yellow, watery or thin liquid

- Serous fluid is often found in cystic structures, but it can occur in any body cavity.
- *Serous fluid* refers to the production of serum, or to fluids containing serum, such as serous exudates.

Tissues commonly affected

Ovaries

Common etiology

Serous carcinoma, serous cystadenoma

Sample gross description

"The cyst contains approximately 10 ml of clear, **serous fluid**."

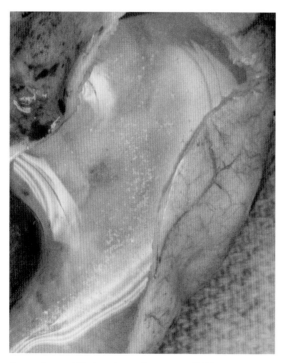

An ovarian cyst that contains clear, serous fluid

Serpiginous

Gross appearance and identification
A lesion or area of interest with a wavy, or snakelike border
- Serpiginous lesions are often ulcers that exhibit healing in 1 portion while continuing to advance in another.

Tissues commonly affected
Skin

Common etiology
Ulcerating lesions

Sample gross description
"Present on the skin surface is a centrally located, light-tan, irregular area, with a **serpiginous** border."

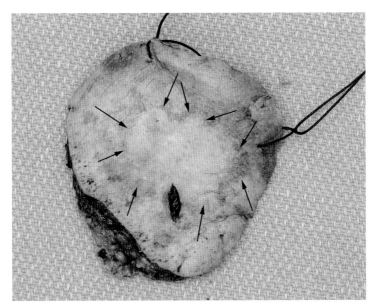

A centrally located lesion (arrows) with a circumferential, serpiginous border

Serrated

Gross appearance and identification
A notched or sawlike edge
- *Serrated* is often used to describe resection margins or the edges of lesions.

Tissues commonly affected
Any

Common etiology
N/A

Sample gross description
"Present on the skin surface is a centrally located dark-tan, roughened lesion, with **serrated** edges."

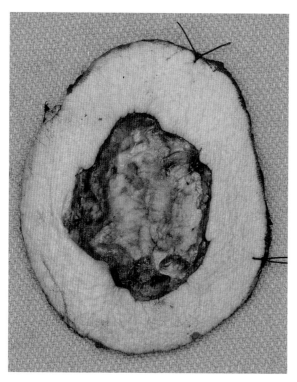

A centrally located lesion with a serrated outer border

Sessile

Gross appearance and identification
Roughened raised areas that have a broad base
- In gross pathology, *sessile* is mostly used to describe polyps in the GI tract.

Tissues commonly affected
GI tract

Common etiology
Sessile polyps

Sample gross description
"Present on the mucosal surface is a tan, **sessile** polyp measuring . . . "

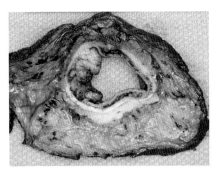

A cross section showing a sessile polyp and its relationship with other bowel layers

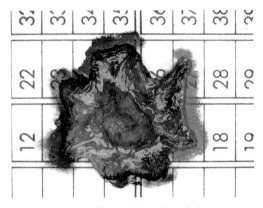

A top-down view of a broad-based sessile lesion on an intestinal mucosa

Sloughed

Gross appearance and identification
An outer layer or covering that is shedding
- *Sloughed* usually refers to a layer or mass of dead tissue separated from surrounding living tissue.
- Skin sloughing results from wounds, sores, or inflammation.

Tissues commonly affected
Skin

Common etiology
Diabetes, trauma, peripheral vascular disease

Sample gross description
"The skin surface at the distal end of the specimen exhibits sharp demarcation from a tan-to-dark-tan congested appearance to a gray-to-white necrotic appearance with areas of **sloughing**."

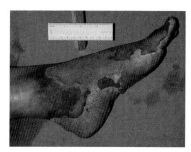

A specimen exhibiting skin sloughing due to tissue necrosis occurring in the distal part of a limb

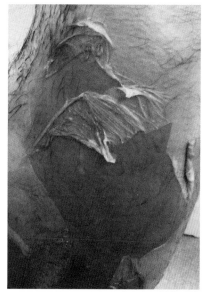

Another example of skin sloughing on a limb

Smooth

Gross appearance and identification
A surface with an even consistency, free from irregularities, roughness, or projections

- In gross specimens, a smooth consistency usually indicates normal pathology.

Tissues commonly affected
Any

Common etiology
N/A

Sample gross description
"The serosal surface appears **smooth** and unremarkable."

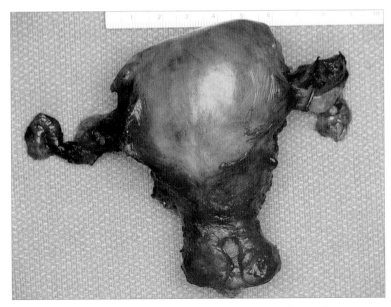

A uterus with a smooth serosal surface, free of any pathologic abnormality

Solid-cystic

Gross appearance and identification
A lesion or area of interest that contains both a solid and cystic component
- If a cyst contains solid areas, it may be a sign that the lesion is precancerous or cancerous.

Tissues commonly affected
Any

Common etiology
Malignant tumors

Sample gross description
"The cut surface of the neoplasm exhibits necrosis with central, **solid-cystic** degeneration containing red serous fluid."

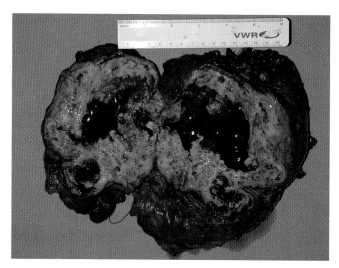

A malignant solid-cystic ovarian lesion that has undergone necrosis, and central, cystic degeneration

Stellate

Gross appearance and identification
A lesion or area of interest that is star shaped
- Stellate lesions exhibit multiple tapering points emanating from a central axis.
- Stellate lesions are often associated with malignant lesions that are infiltrating surrounding normal tissue.

Tissues commonly affected
Breast

Common etiology
Malignant tumors

Sample gross description
"The specimen is sectioned to reveal a firm, **stellate** lesion measuring . . . "

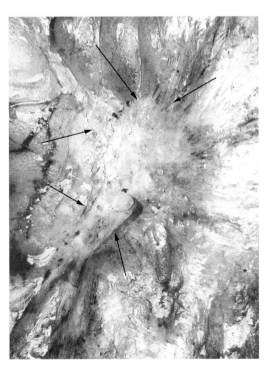

A malignant breast tumor (arrows) with a stellate appearance

Stenotic/strictured

Gross appearance and identification

An abnormal narrowing or contraction of a body passage or opening

- Stenosis or arctation can occur in many areas of the body and usually arises from an underlying pathologic process.

Tissues commonly affected

GI tract, vessels, aorta

Common etiology

Crohn disease, pyloric stenosis, aortic stenosis, pulmonary stenosis

Sample gross description

"The large intestine lumen appears **stenotic/strictured** approximately 6.8 cm from the distal margin due to a focal lesion measuring . . . "

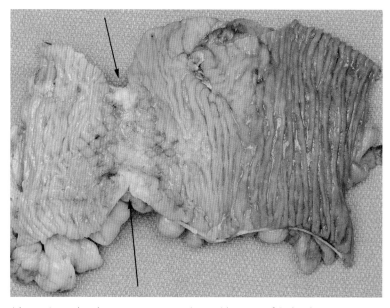

A lumen in a colon that appears stenotic (arrows) because of Crohn disease

Streaked

Gross appearance and identification
Lines defined by a difference in color or texture from surrounding tissue

Tissues commonly affected
Gallbladder

Common etiology
Cholesterolosis

Sample gross description
"The cut surface of the lesion exhibits distinct white **streaking** on a tan-to-red background."

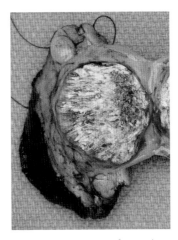

A pilomatrixoma cut surface with diffuse white streaking

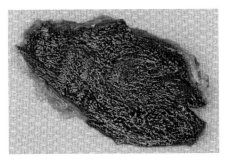

Diffuse yellow streaking on a gallbladder mucosa due to cholesterolosis

Striated

Gross appearance and identification
Thin, regularly alternating lines, bands, stripes, or streaks
- Striations can occur naturally, like muscular bands, or can occur as part of a pathologic process.

Tissues commonly affected
GI tract, skin

Common etiology
Striae gravidarum, atrophic striae

Sample gross description
"The outer surface of the stomach has a distinct **striated** appearance."

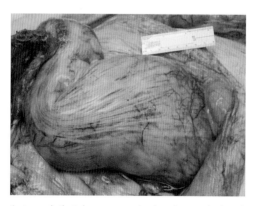

A stomach that shows normal striated muscular bands

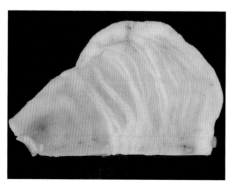

A piece of spinal cord that shows distinct striated white areas on the cut surface

Submucosal

Gross appearance and identification
A lesion or gross area of interest that lies beneath a mucous membrane
- The mucous membrane is a layer of connective tissue beneath the tunica mucosa.

Tissues commonly affected
Bronchi, esophagus, small and large intestines, pharynx, stomach, bladder, uterus

Common etiology
Submucosa hemorrhage, submucosal lipoma

Sample gross description
"The cut surface shows a focal **submucosal** hemorrhagic lesion measuring . . . "

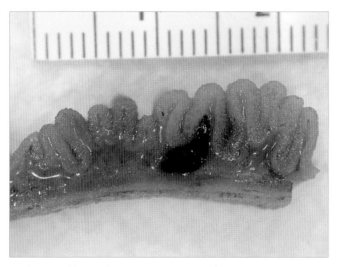

A submucosal hemorrhage in a cross section of intestine

Subserosal

Gross appearance and identification
A lesion or area of interest that lies beneath a serous membrane, such as that of the peritoneum or pericardium

Tissues commonly affected
Bladder, esophagus, gallbladder, small and large intestine, liver, pleura, pericardium, peritoneum, stomach, testes, uterine tubes, uterus

Common etiology
Fibroids

Sample gross description
"Sectioning through the specimen reveals a **subserosal**, white-whorled, well-circumscribed mass measuring . . . "

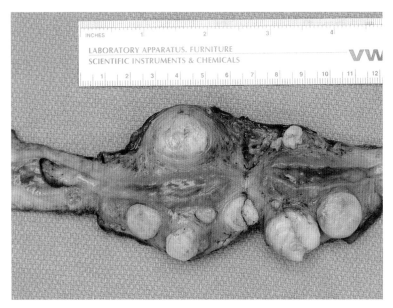

A uterus with a subserosal fibroid (located below the serous membrane)

Symmetrical

Gross appearance and identification
An organ, lesion, or gross abnormality that is the same on either side of a central dividing line

Tissues commonly affected
Any

Common etiology
N/A

Sample gross description
"The specimen consists of a total thyroidectomy specimen with **symmetrical** lobes."

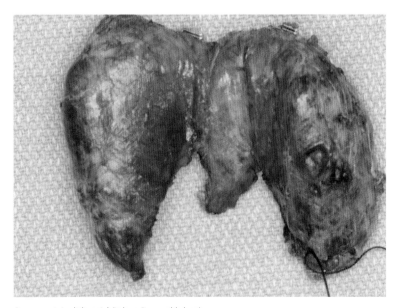

A symmetrical thyroid (it has 2 equal lobes)

Thickened

Gross appearance and identification
Tissue or structures that are thicker than normal, or than adjacent tissue or structures

Tissues commonly affected
Any

Common etiology
Inflammation, tumors

Sample gross description
"Serial sectioning reveals that one-half of the wall appears **thickened** and has a homogeneous light-tan appearance with no clear delineation of the mucosa, muscularis propria, and wall."

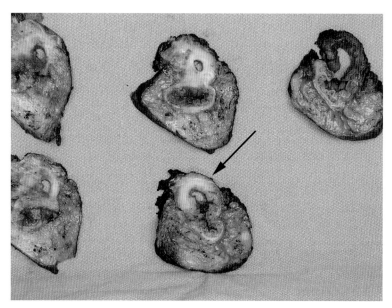

Cross sections of a rectum with a history of rectal cancer: tumor invasion or inflammation due to radiation therapy could account for the thickened portions

Tortuous

Gross appearance and identification
A complexly twisted entity: convoluted and marked by repeated twists, bends, or turns

Tissues commonly affected
Veins, arteries

Common etiology
Hypertension, genetic defects, degenerative vascular diseases (including diabetes mellitus), alterations in blood flow and pressure

- Mild tortuosity is asymptomatic; severe tortuosity can lead to ischemic attack in distal organs.

Sample gross description
"Fetal vessels appear mostly normal with a single **tortuous** vein, eccentrically located, ranging in diameter from…"

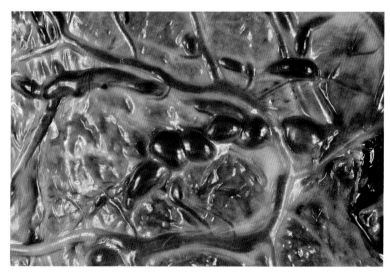

The fetal surface of a placenta with normal arteries and a single tortuous vein

Trabecular

Gross appearance and identification
A thick wall and hypertrophied muscle bundles
- Trabeculation is typically seen in instances of chronic obstruction.

Tissues commonly affected
Gallbladder, bladder, ovaries

Common etiology
Cholecystitis, urinary tract obstruction

Sample gross description
"The inner surface of the cyst is **trabecular**."

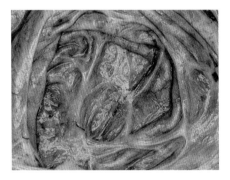

An ovarian inner lining that appears to have a trabecular pattern

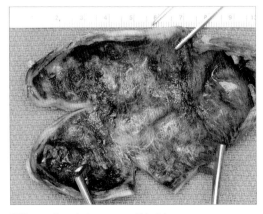

Diffuse trabeculation on a gallbladder mucosa

Translucent

Gross appearance and identification
A substance, lesion, or structure that transmits light, but is not transparent

Tissues commonly affected
Cysts, ovaries, gestational sacs, lung

Common etiology
Spontaneous abortion, molar pregnancy

Sample gross description
"The specimen consists of an ovoid **translucent** cyst with a stalk."

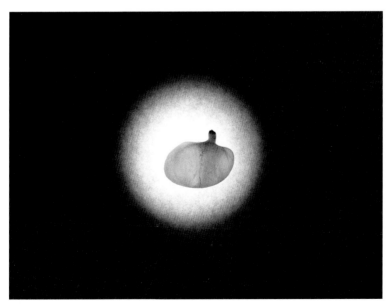

A translucent fluid-filled cyst originating from an ovary

Transparent

Gross appearance and identification
A substance, lesion, or structure that can be seen through

Tissues commonly affected
Ovaries, cysts, gestational sacs, lung

Common etiology
Spontaneous abortion, molar pregnancy

Sample gross description
"The specimen consists of a single, soft, **transparent** cyst measuring . . . "

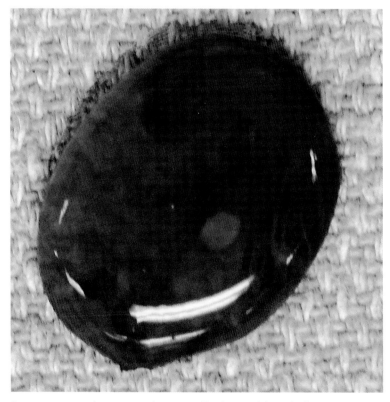

A transparent cyst (you can see the textured background through it)

Ulcerated

Gross appearance and identification
A circumscribed, crater-like lesion
- In ulcers, there is damage where the surface tissue is lost and/or necrotic.
- An ulceration is a local defect, or excavation of the surface, of an organ or tissue, produced by sloughing of necrotic inflammatory tissue.

Tissues commonly affected
Skin, mucous membranes.

Common etiology
Inflammatory, infectious, or malignant processes

Sample gross description
"Present on the mucosa are multiple irregular **ulcerated** lesions."

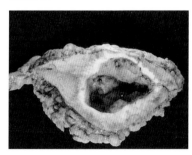

A skin surface with a deep ulceration exposing the underlying subcutaneous tissue

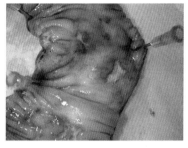

An ulcerated lesion on the mucosal surface of a large bowel, probably due to Crohn disease

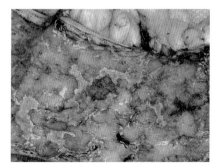

Extensive mucosal ulceration due to ulcerative colitis in a large intestine

Uniform

Gross appearance and identification
A distribution pattern in a lesion or area of interest that is the same throughout (has no distinguishable parts)
- Uniform distribution can indicate a widespread, local metastatic process, or the extent of the disease in question.

Tissues commonly affected
Any

Common etiology
Malignant tumors, inflammatory processes

Sample gross description
"The cut surface of the specimen reveals multiple tan nodules with a **uniform** distribution, which range in size from . . . "

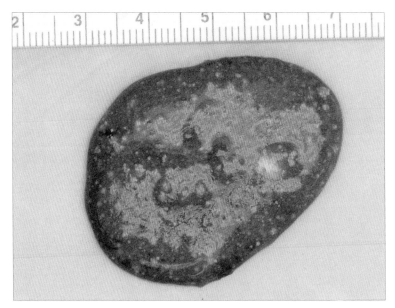

A lesion with speckles that have a uniform distribution

Unilateral

Gross appearance and identification
A lesion or area of interest that is confined within, or that affects, only 1 side of a bilobed or otherwise symmetrical structure

Tissues commonly affected
Any

Common etiology
Ataxia

Sample gross description
"The specimen is sectioned to reveal a single, ill-defined, **unilateral** lesion, which is confined to the left, inferior portion of the lobe, and which measures . . . "

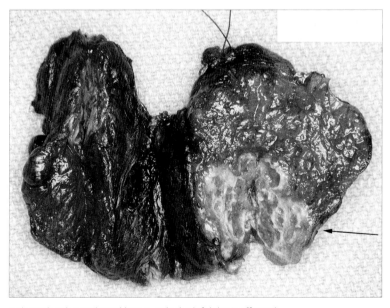

A thyroid with a unilateral lesion: only the left lobe is affected

Variably sized

Gross appearance and identification
Any number of lesions or areas of interest that vary in size

Tissues commonly affected
Ovaries, gallbladder, kidneys

Common etiology
Molar pregnancy, cholelithiasis

Sample gross description
"The specimen is sectioned to reveal a cystic cavity containing multiple translucent cysts of **variable size** ranging from . . . "

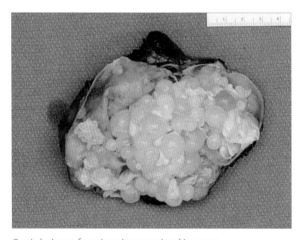

Cystic lesions of varying size contained in a cyst

Variegated

Gross appearance and identification
Tissue or specimens with 2 or more colors, aspects, or features, often with a multifaceted appearance

Tissues commonly affected
Soft tissues, ovary

Common etiology
Malignant or benign tumors

Sample gross description
"The cyst contains a focal, multicystic, tan-and-yellow, **variegated** mass measuring . . . "

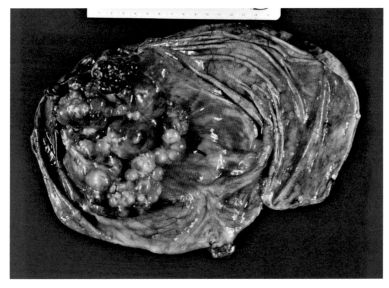

An ovarian cyst that contains a benign tumor with a variegated appearance

Velvety

Gross appearance and identification
A lesion or area of interest that is soft and carpet-like
- A velvety gross appearance is due to the presence of vast numbers of papillae or folds.
- Discolored velvety lesions, especially in the oral cavity, may indicate a pathologic process.

Tissues commonly affected
Mucosal membranes, tongue, oral cavity

Common etiology
Erythroplastic lesions

Sample gross description
"The mucosa appears tan and **velvety**."

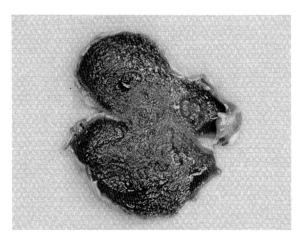

A gallbladder mucosa with a velvety mucosal surface

Vermiform

Gross appearance and identification
Worm-shaped, or resembling a worm, in form
- The appendix of the cecum has a classic vermiform appearance.

Tissues commonly affected
Appendix

Common etiology
N/A

Sample gross description
"The specimen consists of a **vermiform** appendix with attached mesoappendiceal fat."

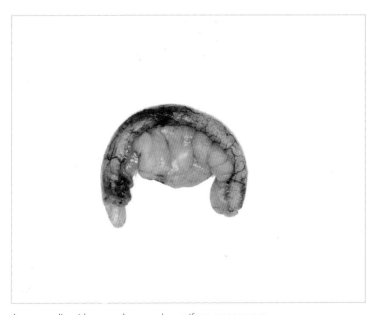

An appendix with a grossly normal vermiform appearance

Verrucous

Gross appearance and identification
A lesion or area of interest that resembles a wart or with wart-like elevations
- Verrucous lesions often indicate human papillomavirus (HPV) infection or inflammatory skin conditions.

Tissues commonly affected
Skin

Common etiology
HPV, verrucose dermatitis, verrucose pododermatitis

Sample gross description
"Present on the surface is a single, gray-white **verrucous** lesion measuring . . . "

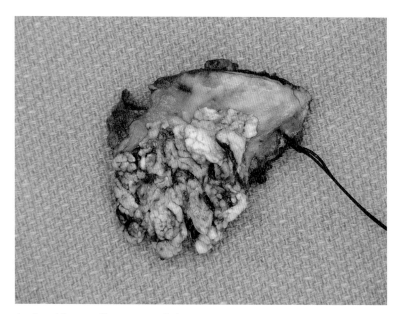

A vulva with a wart-like, verrucous lesion

Vesicle

Gross appearance and identification
A small (< 5 mm in diameter) circumscribed elevated bladder or sac
- Vesicles are known as small blisters.

Tissues commonly affected
Skin, serosal surfaces

Common etiology
Dermatitis, allergic reactions, chicken pox, herpes, autoimmune disease

Sample gross description
"Present on the serosal surface is a single, soft, translucent **vesicle** measuring . . . "

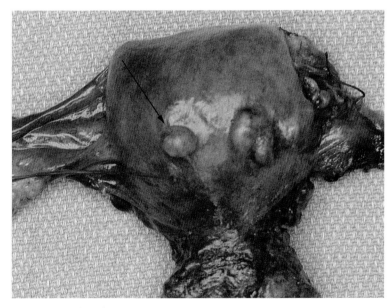

A vesicle (arrow) on the uterine serosa

Well-healed

Gross appearance and identification
A lesion or area of interest that has returned to normal or almost normal appearance

- In gross pathology, *well-healed* is often used to describe areas of previous surgery as compared to areas of more recent surgery.

Tissues commonly affected
Skin

Common etiology
Previous surgery

Sample gross description
"Present on the skin surface is a single, linear, **well-healed** scar, which extends in a superior to inferior direction starting at the proximal margin and which measures . . . "

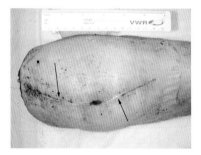

An amputated leg with a well-healed linear scar (arrows) on the skin surface—a sign of previous surgery

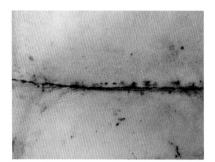

A well-healed incision

Whorled

Gross appearance and identification
A lesion or area of interest with tissue that is curled or wound in concentric rings or spirals

Tissues commonly affected
Uterus

Common etiology
Leiomyoma, leiomyosarcoma

Sample gross description
"The specimen is bisected to reveal a white, **whorled**, well-circumscribed cut surface."

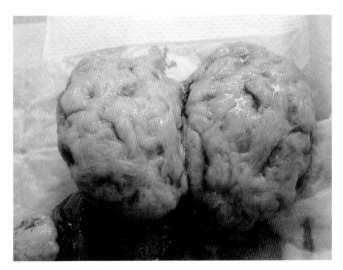

A leiomyoma (fibroid) with a typical whorled appearance on its cut surface

Wrinkled

Gross appearance and identification
Small furrows, ridges, or creases on a normally smooth surface

- In gross pathology, specimens often exhibit wrinkling because of postsurgical tissue contraction and formalin fixation.

Tissues commonly affected
Skin, hernia sacs, cysts

Common etiology
Tissue contraction, formalin fixation

Sample gross description
"The outer surface of the cyst appears gray-tan and **wrinkled**."

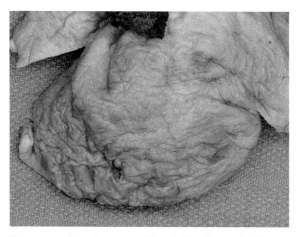

The outer surface of an ovary with wrinkling due to shrinkage from formalin fixation

Index

M

macronodular, 98

macule, 99

malabsorption, gaseous, 72

malignant lesions, puckered, 131

malignant neoplasms, pushing, 135

malignant processes, ulcerated, 163

malignant skin lesions, coalesced, 27

malignant tumors
  bosselated, 16
  caseous, 20
  degeneration, 35
  diffuse, 39
  heterogeneous, 77
  infiltrated, 84
  invasive, 89
  inverted, 90
  perforated, 124
  segmental, 141
  solid-cystic, 150
  stellate, 151
  uniform, 164

mammillated, 100

mastectomy specimens
  ellipse, 46
  peau d'orange, 122

mediastinal lymph nodes, anthracotic pigment, 7

melanocytic nevus, pigmented, 126

melanoma
  fungating, 70
  pigmented, 126

meningococcemia, petechia, 125

mesothelioma, plaque, 127

metastatic lesions, multifocal, 106

metastatic tumors, fractured, 68

miliary, 101

miliary tuberculosis, miliary, 101

molar pregnancies
  botryoid, 17

translucent, 161

transparent, 162

variably sized, 166

mottled, 102

mouth, pedunculated polyp, 123

mucinous, 103

mucinous breast lesions, mucinous, 103

mucinous cyst adenocarcinoma, mucinous, 103

mucinous cystadenoma
  fluid-filled, 66
  mucinous, 103

mucoperiosteum perforation, fenestrated, 57

mucosa, blister, 15

mucosal membrane
  pigmented, 126
  velvety, 168

mucosal surfaces
  macronodular, 98
  macule, 99
  mammillated, 100
  papillate, 119

mucous membranes
  annular/circinate, 6
  papule, 120
  pedunculated polyp, 123
  petechia, 125
  ulcerated, 163

mucous plugs, atelectatic, 10

multicystic, 104

multifaceted, 105

multifocal, 106

multifocal breast cancer, multifocal, 106

multifocal disease, coalesced, 27

multilobular, 107

multilobular osteomas and chondromas, multilobular, 107

multiparous, 108

mummified, 109

muscular dystrophy, atrophic, 11

subserosal, 156
periorbital region, hairy, 75
peripheral edema, edematous, 45
peripheral vascular disease
    mummified, 109
    sloughed, 148
peritoneal cavity, bile-stained, 13
peritoneal surfaces
    exudate, 55
    granulated, 73
peritoneum
    serosal, 143
    subserosal, 156
peritonitis
    exudate, 55
    granulated, 73
petechia, 125
pharynx, submucosal, 155
pigmented, 126
pilar cysts, cystic, 33
pimples, papule, 120
pitting edema, depressed, 38
plaque, 127
pleura
    gaseous, 72
    serosal, 143
    subserosal, 156
pleural cavity, plaque, 127
pneumothorax, gaseous, 72
pollution, anthracotic pigment, 7
polycystic kidney disease
    bilateral, 12
    multicystic, 104
polycystic ovaries, multicystic, 104
polyps, botryoid, 17
postsurgical complications,
    adhesion, 5
protruding, 128
pseudocyst, 129
pseudomembranous colitis,
    plaque, 127
pseudomyxoma peritonei,
    mucinous, 103
pseudopolyp, 130

psoriasis
    plaque, 127
    scaled, 140
puckered, 131
pulmonary edema
    edematous, 45
    fluid-filled, 66
pulmonary embolism, bilateral, 12
pulmonary nodules, ill-defined,
    80
pulmonary stenosis, stenotic/
    strictured, 152
pultaceous/sebaceous material, 132
purulent/suppurating, 133
pus, 134
pushing, 135
pyloric stenosis, stenotic/
    strictured, 152

R
raised, 136
rash
    macronodular, 98
    macule, 99
rectal cancer, protruding, 128
renal calculi, calculus, 19
renal nodule, nodule, 112
reniform, 137
reproductive tract, fistula, 62
rheumatoid nodule, nodule, 112
roughened, 138
ruptured, 139

S
sarcoidosis, annular/circinate, 6
sarcoma
    fleshy, 65
    homogeneous, 78
    multilobular, 107
sarcoma botryoides, botryoid, 17
satellite nodule, nodule, 112
scaled, 140
scarring, linear, 95
schistosomiasis, pseudopolyp, 130

About the Authors

Christopher Horn, MSc, PA(ASCP)^{CM} (CCCPA-CCCAP) is a clinical lecturer in the Department of Pathology and Laboratory Medicine at the University of Calgary and a pathologists' assistant at Alberta Precision Laboratories, where he has performed surgical gross dissection and autopsy services since 1999. He is a past recipient of the Athabasca University Rising Star Award and the Lloyd A. Kennedy Pathologists' Assistant Award, presented by the Canadian Association of Pathologists.

Christopher Naugler, MD, FRCPC, is a professor of pathology and laboratory medicine at the University of Calgary, and associate dean of undergraduate medical education at the Cumming School of Medicine. He is the author of *Lab Literacy for Canadian Doctors*, coauthor of *Lab Literacy for Doctors*, author of *Strategies for the MCCQE Part II: Mastering the Clinical Skills Exam in Canada*, and co-author of *Clinical Skills Review*, all published by Brush Education.

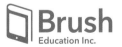

To see all medical and health science resources available from Brush Education, please go to:

www.brusheducation.ca